Edited by E.I. Hernández-Jiménez, E.M. Rakhanskaya

LASER EPILATION AND HAIR REMOVAL
IN COSMETIC DERMATOLOGY & SKINCARE PRACTICE

Cosmetics & Medicine Publishing

Author/Editor:
Elena I. Hernández-Jiménez, *Ph.D.*

Editor:
Ekaterina M. Rakhanskaya, *M.D.* Neurologists, radiation safety specialist

Contributors:
Vera I. Albanova, *M.D., Ph.D., Prof.* Dermatologist
Natalya G. Kalashnikova, *M.D.* Surgeon, dermatologist, laser therapist

LASER EPILATION AND HAIR REMOVAL IN COSMETIC DERMATOLOGY AND SKINCARE PRACTICE

Removing unwanted hair is one of the most requested treatments in modern aesthetic medicine. Many tools are available for this purpose, ranging from those that clients can use on their own, which have a short-term effect, to high-tech devices such as lasers and IPL that offer long-term hair removal. The choice of technique depends on the needs and capabilities of the patient, as well as on the qualifications and expertise of the specialist from whom they seek assistance. The higher the specialist's qualifications, the greater the chances of achieving a lasting effect.

To provide professionals with maximum information on unwanted hair removal, this book covers a comprehensive range of issues crucial for truly effective and safe depilation and epilation procedures. What features of hair structure and growth should be considered when choosing a hair removal technique? How do depilation and epilation techniques function? What outcomes can be anticipated from the procedures, and how can one achieve the best results? Why are lasers and IPL devices considered the "gold standard" for removing unwanted hair? What should one expect from them, and how can they be appropriately used in each case? What complications may arise from the procedures, and how can they be avoided? All this and much more, described in detail, clearly, and engagingly, will be covered in our new book. After all, it is only by understanding what we are working with and the possibilities certain tools offer that we can solve a problem in the best possible way.

The book will be helpful to all specialists who deal with the problem of unwanted hair removal — those who have been practicing for a long time and those who are just starting. In addition, it will be of interest to everyone trying to find the best option for removing unwanted hair for themselves.

ISBN 978-1-970196-30-6 (paperback)
ISBN 978-1-970196-50-4 (hardcover)
ISBN 978-1-970196-33-7 (eBook – Adobe PDF)
ISBN 978-1-970196-34-4 (eBook – ePUB)

Author/Editor

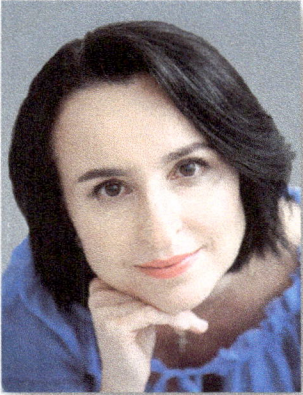

Elena I. Hernández-Jiménez, *Ph.D.*

Biophysicist, scientific journalist

Editor-in-chief of Cosmetics and Medicine Publishing

Member of the International Society of Applied Corneotherapy (I.A.C.); Chair of the I.A.C. Executive Board (May, 2019 – May, 2025)

Author and co-author of numerous publications in professional magazines, co-author and editor of the book series *Fundamentals of Cosmetic Dermatology & Skincare, Cosmetic Dermatology & Skincare Practice, Cosmetic Chemistry for Dermatology & Skincare Specialists* and others

Speaker at international conferences, author of training seminars and webinars for professionals in the field of skincare

Professional interests: biology and physiology of the skin, skin permeability, cosmetic chemistry, anti-age medicine, physiotherapy in dermatology and aesthetic medicine, skin analysis and imaging

Table of Contents

PART I
HAIR AS A THERAPEUTIC TARGET

PART III

COMMON COMPLICATIONS OF HAIR REMOVAL

(*V.I. Albanova*)

List of abbreviations

ALH   — acquired localized hypertrichosis
CMC   — cell membrane complex
Da   — Dalton
DLQI   — Dermatology Life Quality Index
ELOS   — ELectro-Optical Synergy
Er:YAG   — erbium-doped yttrium aluminum garnet laser
ESLD   — European Society of Laser Dermatology
FDA   — Food and Drug Administration
FP   — fibrillar protein
HF   — hair follicle
HFS   — high-frequency sonophoresis
HLA   — hypertrichosis lanuginosa acquisita
Hz   — hertz
IPL   — intense pulsed light
IR   — infrared light
ISAPS   — International Society of Aesthetic Plastic Surgery
LFS   — low-frequency sonophoresis
LTR   — localized transport region
MC1R   — melanocortin 1 receptor
Nd:YAG   — neodymium-doped yttrium aluminum garnet laser
Nd:YAP   — neodymium-doped yttrium aluminum perovskite laser
NSAIDs   — non-steroidal anti-inflammatory drugs
PCOS   — polycystic ovary syndrome
pH   — potential of hydrogen
PUVA   — psoralen plus ultraviolet-A radiation
QSw   — Q-Switched
RF   — radiofrequency
TNF-α   — tumor necrosis factor alpha
TRT   — thermal relaxation time
UV   — ultraviolet
VAS   — Visual Analog Scale

Introduction

Unwanted hair is a significant, yet often underestimated, aesthetic defect that is normal physiologically, but may be perceived as a problem by the patient. In some cases, excessive hair growth is a symptom of disease. Researchers have noted that individuals suffering from hirsutism — a disorder manifesting as excessive hair growth — have a higher risk of depression and other psychiatric disorders (Canat M.M. et al., 2023). However, the degree of reduction in the quality of life and social disadaptation experienced by patients may not correspond to the severity of excessive hair growth. Patients with a mild degree of hirsutism may develop severe depression, while in others, even pronounced growth of unwanted hair does not cause a negative perception of their body and social limitations. Subjective factors — beauty standards accepted in a particular society, religious and socio-cultural norms, as well as psychological characteristics of the patient — play a decisive role in the attitude toward the problem of unwanted hair and the perceived need for its elimination.

According to the statistics compiled by the International Society of Aesthetic Plastic Surgery (ISAPS) for 2022, removal of unwanted hair ranks among the top three most popular non-surgical aesthetic correction procedures for women, surpassed only by botulinum toxin and hyaluronic acid injections (Triana L. et al., 2024). In 2022, unwanted hair removal procedures accounted for 9.5% of all non-surgical procedures worldwide. They were most in demand in the USA, Japan, and India, and least in Germany and Iran. Notably, in southern European countries, the frequency of procedures was several times higher than in northern and western countries. In Greece, for example, 15 times more procedures were performed to remove unwanted hair than in the UK. The apparent reason for this pattern lies in the ethnic characteristics of hair growth, climate — specifically, how long areas of the body remain covered by clothing throughout the year — along with the widespread public attitude toward the issue of unwanted hair.

Regardless, approximately 2 million unwanted hair removal procedures were performed in 2022, reflecting a 96% increase from 2018. This figure underscores the significant demand for unwanted hair removal.

This book will discuss in detail the normal and pathological physiology of hair growth and the various hair removal techniques.

Part I

Hair as a therapeutic target

Chapter 1
Hair structure

What we refer to as hair in everyday life is actually just the outer part that protrudes above the skin surface. Likewise, when discussing hair removal, we usually mean removing this visible part — the hair shaft. However, to "remove hair permanently" or at least for a prolonged period, the focus should be on the inner part of the hair — the hair follicle (HF). The HF is located beneath the skin and hidden from view, and it is where the processes that enable hair growth take place. Therefore, no matter how much we remove the shaft, if the follicle is preserved, hair growth will continue. To understand how to destroy the HF, we must have a good knowledge of hair anatomy and physiology.

1.1. Hair under the microscope

Hair is an appendage of the skin. This is important to remember because they have much in common, from the structure to the peculiarities of growth and development.

The outer layer of the skin, the epidermis, consists of keratinocytes at various stages of development. Their maturation process ends when they lose their nucleus and turn into dead, keratin-filled corneocytes, which provide protection from external influences and moisture loss. Under the epidermis is the dermis, where the skin appendages are located, including hair follicles and sebaceous and sweat glands. The nails, appendages located on the distal phalanges of the fingers, also grow from the dermis.

Finally, the deepest layer of skin, located beneath the dermis, is the hypodermis, which consists of adipose tissue interspersed with connective tissue septa. Blood vessels and nerve fibers traversing the hypodermis penetrate the dermis, where they transform into

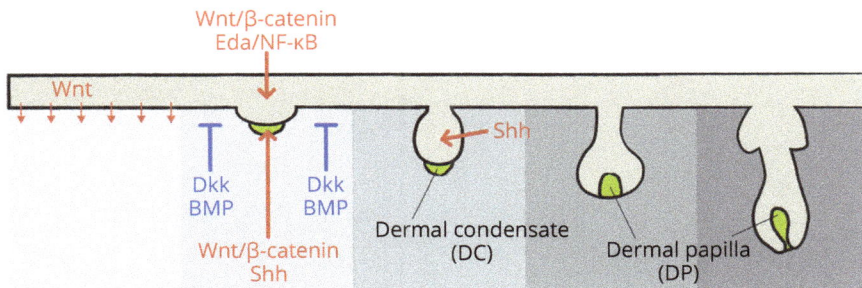

Figure I-1-1. During embryonic development, the skin epithelium undergoes differentiation to form hair follicles. The epithelial cells in the epidermis thicken to create a structure called a placode, while mesenchymal cells in the dermis gather beneath it to form a dermal condensate (DC) (adapted from Park S., 2022)

blood capillaries and nerve endings, respectively, while interacting with the appendages. The formation of hair follicles begins in the fourth month of embryonic development and is governed by the interaction between the dermal and epidermal components (**Fig. I-1-1**).

Anatomically, the hair is divided into two parts:

- Inner part (hair root) — located under the skin and produces hair fibers
- Outer part (hair shaft or hair fiber) — located above the skin, and is a strong and flexible fiber

1.1.1. Hair root

Hair root is covered by epithelial root sheaths (together, they form the hair follicle) and then by a connective tissue dermal sheath (external and internal). Adjacent to the hair follicle are the sweat and sebaceous glands (**Fig. I-1-2**).

The hair root is the living part of the hair hidden deep within the skin. It has upper and lower segments. The upper segment contains auxiliary elements — the sebaceous gland and the muscle that lifts the hair. The lower segment — the hair follicle, a unique multi-layered structure that produces hair fibers — is in the lower segment, which is shaped like a bulb.

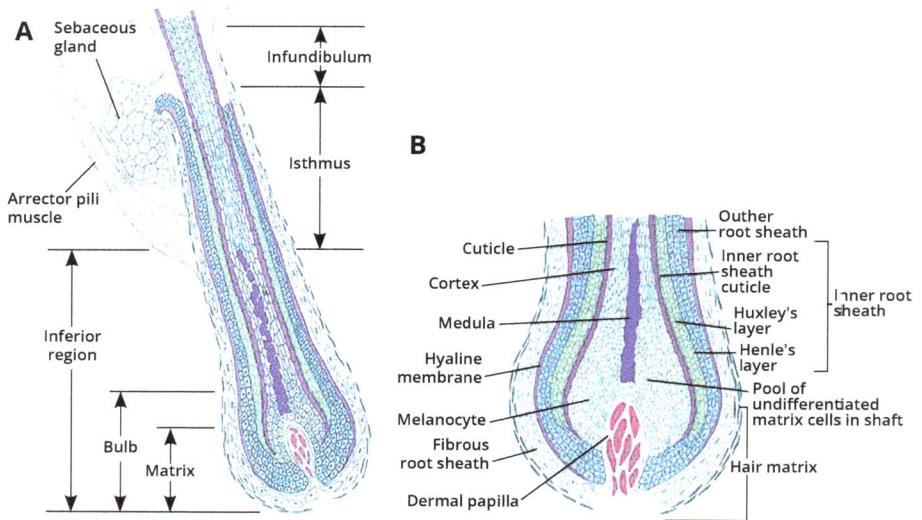

Figure I-1-2. Hair root: A — key components; B — hair bulb

The follicle of an adult human contains two main types of cells involved in hair formation during embryogenesis: fibroblast-like cells (mesenchyme) and epidermal cells (ectoderm). The dermal part of the hair follicle consists of specialized fibroblast-like cells of the dermal papilla and the fibrous root sheath. There are up to nine types of epidermal cells: cells of the medulla, cortex, inner and outer layers of the bulb, and Henle's and Huxley's layers. This cellular complex also includes melanocytes, which are of ectodermal origin.

The cells of the dermal follicle — keratinocytes, melanocytes, and fibroblasts — are at different stages of differentiation and function depending on the stage of the hair lifecycle (see below). Highly differentiated cells are involved in hair fiber production. Undifferentiated stem cells form a cellular reserve and are dormant for the time being. When the follicle transitions from the resting phase to the growth phase, some of these stem cells are activated with subsequent division and maturation. In addition, they are involved in healing and skin repair after damage (Huang S. et al., 2021; Lin X. et al., 2022). Two main stem cell niches are identified in the hair follicle. One is in the bulge area at the junction of the external root sheath and the muscle that lifts the hair, and the other is located inside the bulb.

The hair bulb acts as the factory that produces the hair shaft. Below, connective tissue with blood capillaries extends into the hair follicle — the dermal papilla. This structure is one of the key centers for regulating hair growth, and beneath it lies a niche of stem cells.

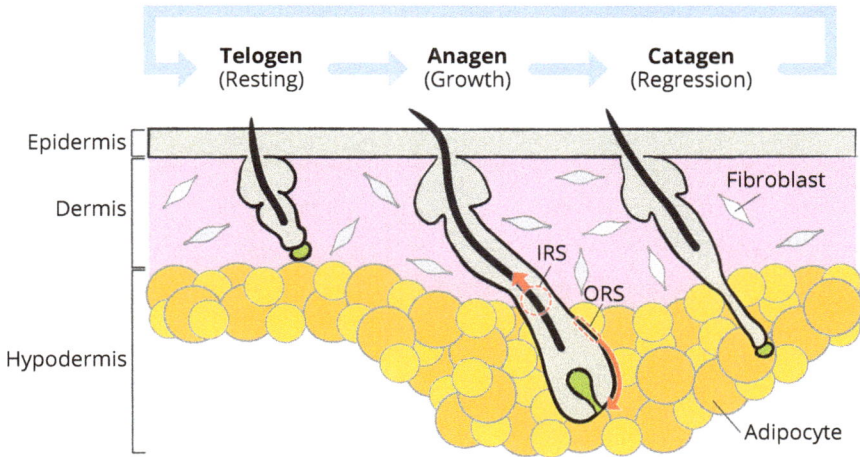

Figure I-1-3. Immersion of the hair follicle in the hypodermis during the growth stage. IRS — inner root sheath, ORS — outer root sheath (adapted from Park S., 2022)

Looking ahead, **the main targets of hair growth prevention treatments are stem cells, which are the cellular reserve of the hair follicle, and the dermal papilla, which provides nourishment**.

The follicle is embedded in a layer of subcutaneous fatty tissue. Researchers have observed an accumulation of fat cells (adipocytes) around awake normal follicles that actively produce healthy hair and their relative scarcity around dormant follicles (**Fig. I-1-3**). From this, it has been concluded that adipocytes are essential for supporting hair follicle function (Li K.N., Tumbar T., 2021; Park S., 2022). With age, this layer thins in most areas of the body. Factors that inhibit hair growth, such as chemotherapy or starvation, also reduce the subcutaneous fat.

Continuous hair growth occurs due to the division (proliferation) of cells located on the hyaline basal membrane, which separates the inner part of the follicle from the outer connective tissue sheath. Cell detachment from the basal membrane signals the onset of maturation (differentiation), leading to cell death: maturing cells gradually lose their nuclei, fill with keratin, and alter their shape.

Due to continuous cell division within the follicle, pressure is created that forces keratinized cells to move upward at a rate of approximately 0.3–0.4 mm per day, thus ensuring hair shaft growth.

1.1.2. Hair shaft

A cross-section of the hair shaft shows two zones, a thin and dense sheath (cuticle) covering a relatively loose interior (cortex). In some hairs, another zone (medulla) is visible at the center of the cortex. Thus, the hair shaft consists of two or three layers (**Fig. I-1-4**).

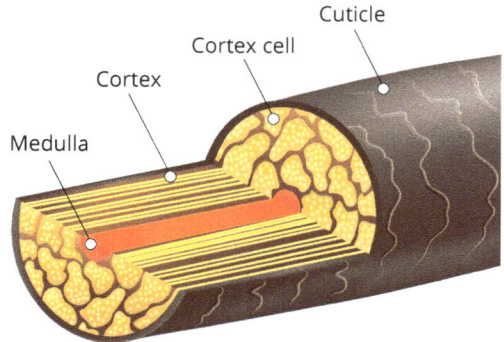

Figure I-1-4. Layers of the hair shaft (photo by Freepik)

There are no living cells in the hair shaft, only dead cells. They are bound together by a lipid–protein structure called the **cell membrane complex (CMC)** (Yang F.C. et al., 2014). The composition and structure of CMC differ in various layers, but its function is universal: CMC is the glue responsible for the integrity of the hair fiber. The mechanical properties of the hair fiber — strength and flexibility — largely depend on it. If it is damaged (e.g., by overly energetic brushing), the hair becomes brittle, begins to split, and becomes electrified (Coderch L. et al., 2023).

Cuticle: the protective sheath of the stem

The cuticle consists of 6 to 10 layers of overlapping scales. These scales are transparent, colorless, and repel water. They have an oblong shape, measuring 0.2 to 0.5 µm in thickness, about 0.3 µm in width, and up to 100 µm in length, and are arranged like tiles.

One cuticle cell covers 1/3 to 1/2 of the hair shaft circumference. The spaces between the cuticle cells are filled with CMC. The CMC consists of beta layers (lipids) that are covered by a delta layer (protein). The CMC is 0.04 to 0.06 µm thick. Hair dye and other hair products penetrate the hair through the CMC.

Chemical and electrostatic bonds formed between keratin proteins in different layers of hair — primarily covalent disulfide bonds (the strongest), along with ionic and hydrogen interactions — help the hair shaft maintain the shape of a tightly compressed twine.

During coloring and bleaching, these bonds are broken, which also negatively impacts the mechanical properties of the hair.

The cuticle's structure resembles the *stratum corneum*, which is also composed of keratin scales — corneocytes (though their shape is different — hexagonal) — glued by a lipid substance (in the *stratum corneum*, this is called a lipid barrier).

The cuticle is the toughest part of the hair, protecting its interior.

Cortex: the layer responsible for the mechanical properties of the hair

Beneath the cuticle is the cortical layer, the cortex, composed of cortical cells with a diameter of 1–5 µm and a length of 50–100 µm. CMC is found between the cortex cells, but its chemical composition and structure differ from the CMC of the cuticle (Robbins C.R., 2012).

Cortical cells are aligned along the hair fiber. Their basic structures consist of tightly adhering keratin macrofibrils. Each macrofibril is a collection of microfibrils, and the spaces between them are filled with a hydrophilic matrix (**Figs. I-1-5 – I-1-7**). The main component of this matrix is amorphous keratin. Additionally, the matrix contains a large amount of melanin pigment, amino acids, polypeptides, nucleic acids, and minerals. When perming, bleaching, and coloring hair, the matrix is damaged, negatively impacting the condition of the hair.

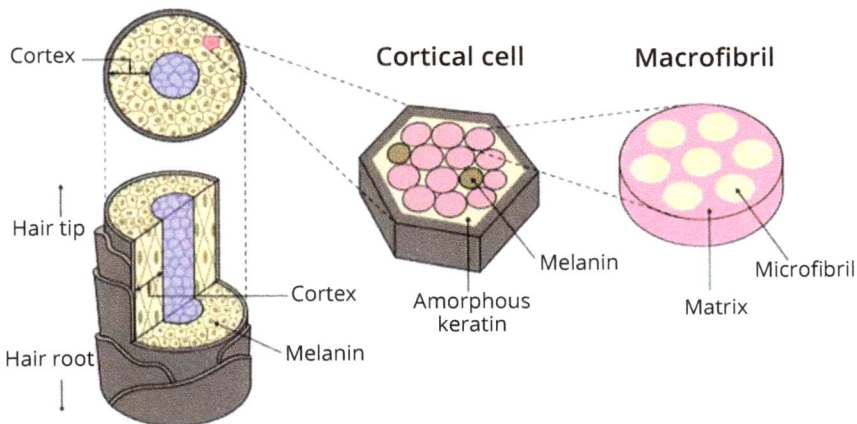

Figure I-1-5. Structure of the hair cortex: general plan
(Keyence Corporation of America; www.keyence.com)

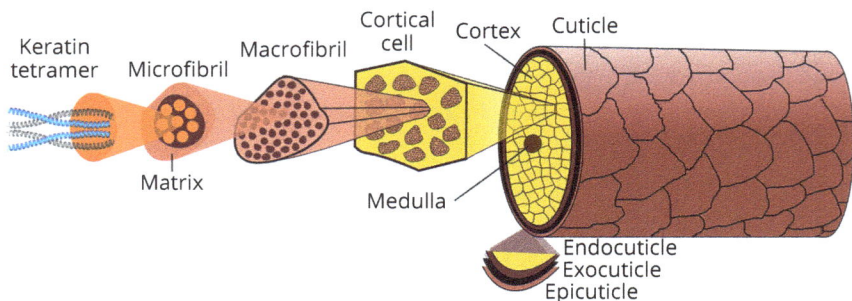

Figure I-1-6. Organization of the keratin fibrils in the hair shaft (adapted from Cruz C.F. et al., 2016)

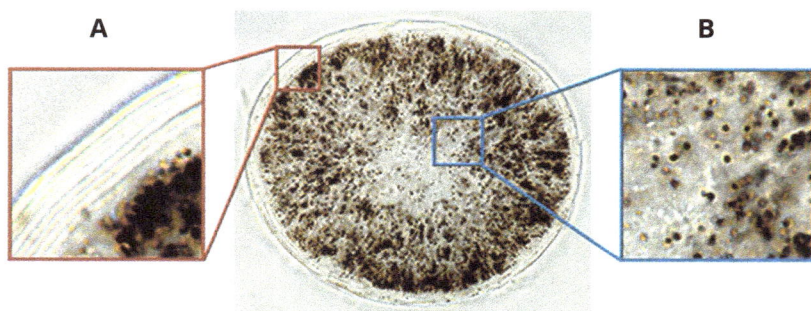

Figure I-1-7. Cross-section of human hair. Imaging method: Brightfield. Objective lens 100× (oil immersion). A — laminar structure of the cuticle; B — melanin found across the cortex (Keyence Corporation of America; www.keyence.com)

Cortex gives the shaft flexibility and strength, and is also responsible for hair color.

Medulla: insulating properties of the hair

Some hairs have a medulla beneath the cortex, which has many cavities. In animals, the medulla is well developed — the presence of air inside the hair shaft reduces its thermal conductivity. Such hair serves as reliable thermal insulation and protects the body from environmental temperature fluctuations. In humans, the medulla is present in stiff hair (especially gray hair).

1.2. Hair lifecycle

The life of an individual hair is cyclical and consists of a growth phase (anagen), an intermediate phase (catagen), and a loss phase (telogen) (**Table I-1-1**; **Fig. I-1-8**).

Typically, the number of hair follicles at different stages is balanced, ensuring that each individual's hair coverage remains relatively constant (**Fig. I-1-8**).

Table I-1-1. Hair lifecycle

PHASE	DURATION	WHAT'S GOING ON
Anagen (growth phase)	2–8 years	The cells in the follicle divide intensively. Hair growth rate averages at about 1 cm per month (0.5 to 3 cm) and varies from season to season (for example, hair grows faster in winter). Pigment is actively produced in this phase, but this process slows down with age.
Catagen (intermediate phase)	A few weeks	Hair growth stops and no pigment is formed. The follicle gradually shrinks in size and moves towards the skin surface.
Telogen (shedding or resting phase)	3 months on average	During this period, a hair may fall out spontaneously or as a result of light effort. Spontaneous hair loss usually occurs when a new hair begins to grow under the old hair.

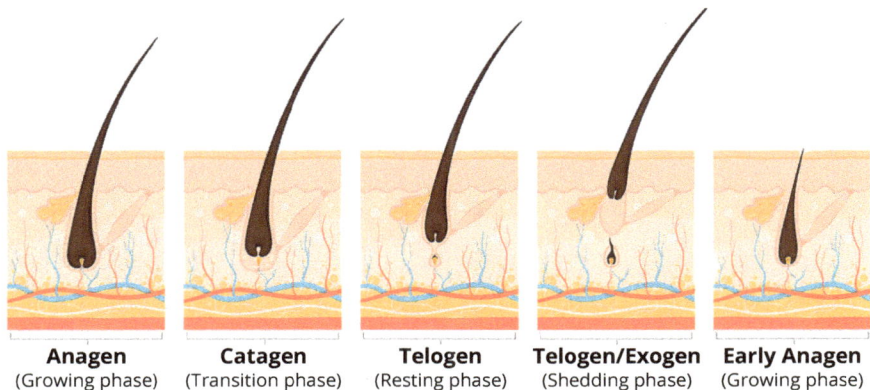

| **Anagen** (Growing phase) | **Catagen** (Transition phase) | **Telogen** (Resting phase) | **Telogen/Exogen** (Shedding phase) | **Early Anagen** (Growing phase) |

Figure I-1-8. The hair lifecycle (image by Paper Teo/Shutterstock)

Over the years, the quality of hair on different parts of the body changes (**Table I-1-2**), showing a gradual transition from one type of hair to another and the appearance of hair where none originally existed. This natural process is regulated by the endocrine system and differs between men and women (**Fig. I-1-9**).

The phase of the hair, whether in anagen or telogen, is crucial at the time of epilation, as **only anagen hair is sensitive to physical treatments**.

The percentage of hair follicles in the anagen phase can vary across different parts of the body and is also influenced by external and internal factors (**Fig. I-1-10**) (Natarelli N. et al., 2023).

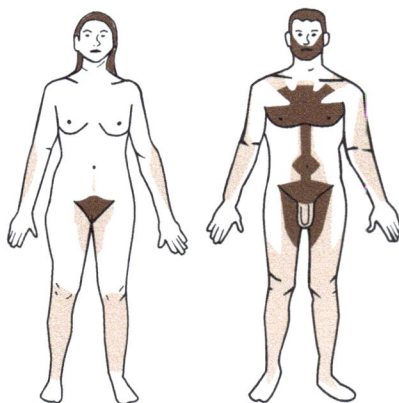

Figure I-1-9. Hair cover in women and men: growth zones of pubescent hair are indicated in light brown, terminal hairs in dark brown

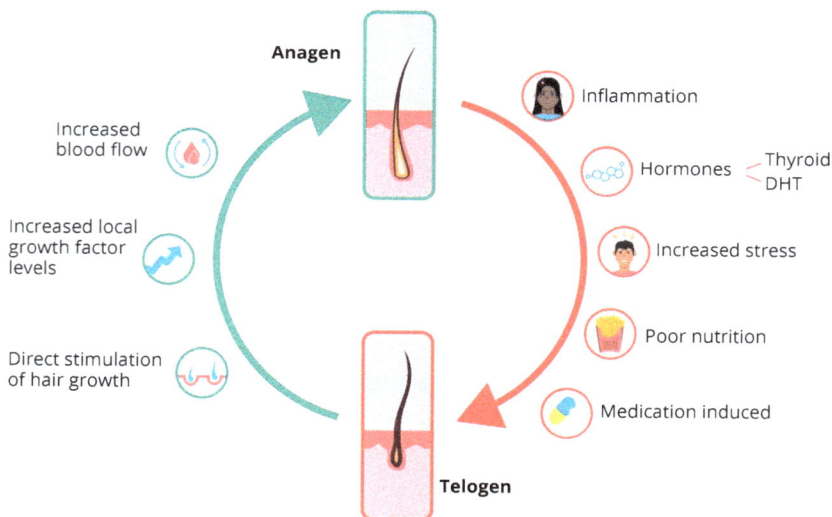

Figure I-1-10. Schematic diagram of the hair growth cycle and the factors that may influence a transition from anagen to telogen vs. telogen to anagen phase (adapted from Natarelli N. et al., 2023)

Table I-1-2. Hair in different periods of human life

HAIR TYPE	PERIODS OF HUMAN LIFE			
	FETUS / NEWBORN	CHILDHOOD	ADULTHOOD	OLD AGE
Lanugo Thin, of equal length, colorless. Grows synchronously and evenly over the entire body.	Appears in the 3rd month of fetal development. At 36 weeks of fetal life, it falls out.	Absent	Absent	Absent
Vellus Short (1–2 cm) in pubescence, almost without pigment. It grows from small follicles located in the upper layer of the dermis.	At birth, there's some hair on the scalp.	It grows all over the body and on the head.	A little on the scalp; on the body, it is gradually replaced by stiff hairs.	Normally absent. However, in androgenetic alopecia, hair may appear on the parietal part of the head.
Terminal (stiff, long) hair Normal hair	At birth, hairs are present on the scalp, eyebrows, and eyelashes.	Growing on the scalp, eyebrows, and eyelashes.	Gradually replaces downy body hair and appears in the armpits and pubic area. The hair shaft becomes thicker and longer. In men, growth appears on the chin and neck.	The anagen phase tends to shorten. Hair becomes finer and pigment formation decreases. In the elderly, stiff hair tends to grow more abundantly on the face, as well as in the nostrils and ears, while the long scalp hair gradually dies off.

At any given time, approximately 56–76% of facial hair is in the anagen phase (Fernandez-Flores A. et al., 2019).

1.3. Hair color

Hair pigmentation is linked to melanocytes, which are large, sprouting cells that produce the pigment melanin.

During embryonic development, melanocytes do not reach their permanent locations immediately. Initially, all epidermal cells and nerve cells develop from the same embryonic layer — the ectoderm — but while the paths of keratinocyte and nerve cell precursors diverge early, melanocyte precursors (melanoblasts) continue to develop for some time as part of the neural crest. Only by the 6th to 8th week of intrauterine development do they "catch up" with the epithelial (external) ectoderm, penetrating the basal layer of the epidermis and the rudiments of hair follicles (it is assumed that for this purpose they use sprouting into the skin nerve endings as a "funicular"). By the 12th to 13th week, most melanoblasts localize in the epidermis, and a little later "get" to the hair follicles, where they differentiate into melanocytes. Some melanoblasts do not differentiate and are "stored" in the bulge zone as stem cells. There are suggestions that some of these stem cells may remain directly in the dermis (Bismuth K. et al., 2017).

Melanocytes are located at the apex of the hair follicle. During the anagen phase, they can also be found near the hair papilla in the basal layer of the epidermis. Single melanocytes are present in the funnel zone of the hair follicle (*infundibulum*) and within the wall of sebaceous glands (Torres F., 2015).

The substrate for pigment biosynthesis is the amino acid tyrosine. If it is lacking, pigment may be formed from another amino acid, phenylalanine, which can be converted into tyrosine. As a result of a series of complex enzymatic transformations, in which the enzyme tyrosinase plays a significant role, two pigments (brown–black eumelanins and yellow–orange pheomelanin) are formed (**Fig. I-1-11**). Their ratio depends on the genetic program, a variant of the melanocortin 1 receptor (*MC1R*) gene. Both pigments are produced by melanocytes

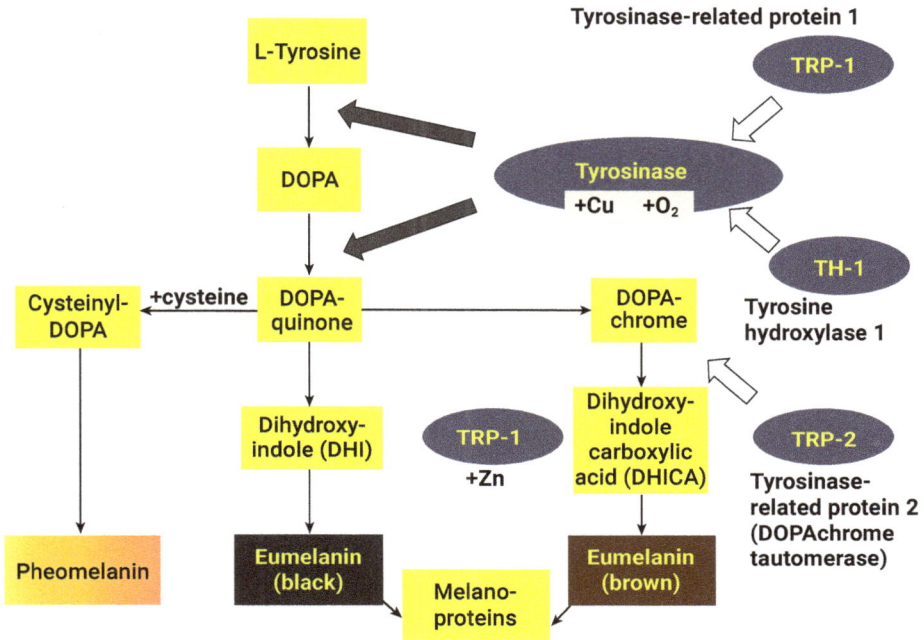

Figure I-1-11. Schematic diagram of melanin synthesis

during the anagen phase, but they have slightly different functions and are packaged differently: mature melanosomes containing eumelanins are ellipsoidal, while pheomelanin is spherical.

In people with red hair, both *MC1R* gene copies are defective, and there is virtually no eumelanin. Eumelanin is also scarce in fair-haired people, in whom defective *MC1R* is present in a heterozygous state. The predominance of pheomelanin in fair-haired people gives the hair a more golden or slightly pinkish hue, while eumelanin gives the hair an ashy or light sandy color.

In all people, regardless of their race, melanocytes synthesize both eumelanin and pheomelanin. However, pheomelanin is synthesized "by default," and the amount of eumelanin is greater in people with a higher phototype. In dark-haired individuals, nearly all melanin is comprised of eumelanin, which is brown or black. At the same time, hair color depends not only on the ratio of melanins but also on their total amount; black hair contains the most melanin. **Fig. I-1-12** shows

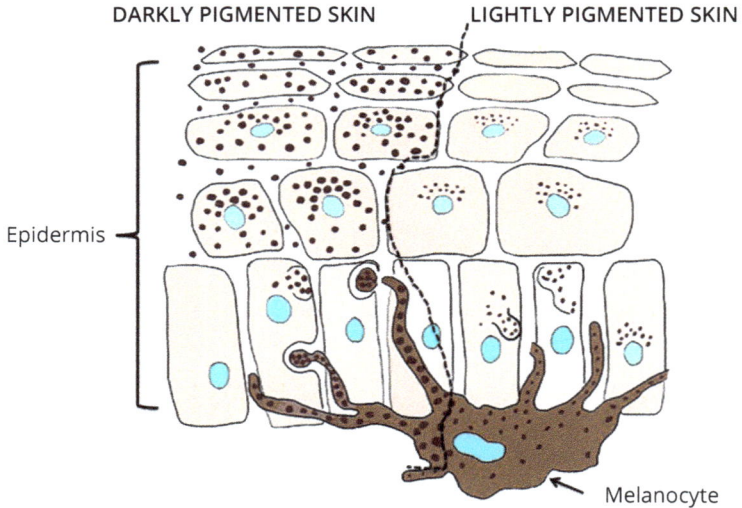

Figure I-1-12. Distribution of melanin in the skin of dark-pigmented and light-skinned individuals (adapted from Adhikari M. et al., 2018)

the distribution of melanin in the skin of dark-skinned and light-skinned individuals — a similar pattern of melanin distribution is observed in dark and light hair.

In graying hair, the number of melanocytes in the basal HF cells decreases; they undergo dystrophy and gradually disappear altogether. That is, there is no melanin in gray hair.

Sometimes the same person can have differently colored hair growing on different parts of the body, such as dark hair on the head and red hair in the beard and mustache area. This phenomenon is called **heterochromia**.

There is a specific correlation between hair color and thickness. Redheads have the thickest hair (up to 100 μm in diameter), blondes have the thinnest hair (50 μm), and brunettes have the average thickness (about 75 μm).

The whole process of melanogenesis takes place intracellularly in special organelles — melanosomes — which are then transferred to the surrounding keratinocytes of the hair follicle by cytoplasmic outgrowths (dendrites). In the hair shaft, melanin is accumulated in the cortical cells.

In the interfollicular epidermis, melanocytes in the basal layer represent 10% of all cells, and each supplies pigment to about 40 keratinocytes (together, the melanocyte and the keratinocytes it serves constitute the so-called melanin unit). In the hair follicle, each melanocyte serves five keratinocytes, and only one in the matrix region. In addition, hair follicle melanocytes are larger than the epidermal ones and have more dendrites (Fernandez-Flores A. et al., 2019).

Melanogenesis in hair follicles, unlike epidermal melanogenesis, closely relates to the phases of the hair lifecycle. In the early anagen phase, melanocyte precursors migrate into the growing hair follicle and begin producing melanin; in middle and late anagen, this process is at its peak activity. At the end of anagen, melanocytes cease pigment production, and their cytoplasmic outgrowths (dendrites) shorten. The enzymes involved in pigment formation become inactive, so no pigment formation occurs during the telogen phase.

As previously mentioned, melanocyte precursors are found within and beneath the bulge zone (Nishimura E.K. et al., 2005). Multipotent stem cells reside in the bulge, serving as the source of melanocytes responsible for skin and hair pigmentation and providing the "hair pigment unit" in each cycle.

1.4. Ethnic characteristics of hair

There are notable differences in the hair structure and properties among different ethnic groups. Studies of ethnic peculiarities of hair chemical composition and structure have allowed researchers to divide them into three main types (Fernandes C. et al., 2023):

- Caucasian
- Negroid
- Mongoloid

The main interethnic differences in the chemical composition of hair relate to fibrillar proteins (FPs) and CMC. The greatest level of FPs is found in hair of the Mongoloid type. CMC is most pronounced in the hair of representatives from the Negroid ethnic group. However, the FP/CMC ratio, which differs significantly among hair types, is

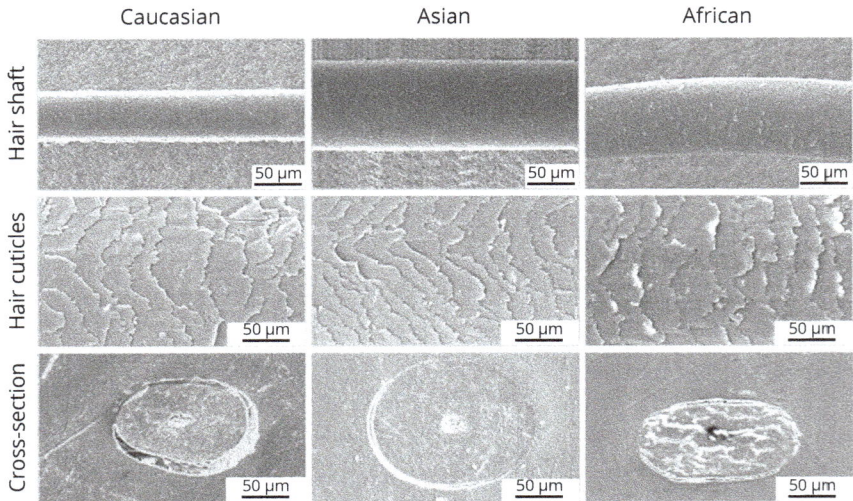

Figure I-1-13. Comparison of hair fiber surface and cross-section from Caucasian, Asian, and African people based on SEM images (adapted from Fernandes C. et al., 2023)

the most informative aspect. Mongoloid type hair is characterized by the highest FP/CMC value, while the lowest value is typical of Negroid hair. This parameter significantly impacts hair properties: the higher FP content compared to CMC, characteristic of Mongoloid hair, may explain its greater strength. Conversely, the low FP content in Negroid hair is believed to contribute to its increased brittleness.

The main distinguishing features of different hair types are the cross-sectional shape and diameter of the hair shaft. Mongoloid hair has a rounded cross-section and a larger diameter (about 100 µm), while Caucasoid hair is usually thinner (about 50 µm in diameter) and slightly elliptical in cross-section. Hair of the Negroid type is elliptical in cross-section and about 80 µm thick, although with greater heterogeneity in diameter than other types. The length of visible cuticle cells varies from 5 to 10 µm, depending on the hair type (**Fig. I-1-13**).

Chapter 2
Diseases accompanied by excessive hair growth

Not only healthy individuals, but also those with excessive hair growth due to a medical condition, may seek removal of unwanted hair. Excessive hair growth can be genetically determined or a result of various diseases and pathological conditions. There are two main forms of excessive hair growth with different causes and clinical features — hirsutism and hypertrichosis.

2.1. Hirsutism

Hirsutism is the term that describes an excessive growth of terminal hair of the male type, occurring in about 5–15% of premenopausal women (Unluhizarci K. et al., 2023). Hirsutism has a significant negative impact on quality of life and causes severe psychological distress.

The main links in the pathogenesis of hirsutism include changes in androgen levels and the ratio of different types of androgens in serum, as well as increased sensitivity of the hair follicle to androgens.

The most common cause of hirsutism is polycystic ovary syndrome (PCOS), accounting for 57.7% of all cases, followed by idiopathic hirsutism (22.6%). Other causes include late congenital adrenal hyperplasia (9.9%), thyroid disease (4.2%), and hyperprolactinemia (rarely presented with isolated hirsutism). Less commonly, hirsutism accompanies pituitary, ovarian, and adrenal tumors. Hirsutism may also be associated with obesity, insulin resistance, diabetes mellitus, hypertension, infertility, and menstrual disorders (Ansari R.T. et al., 2024).

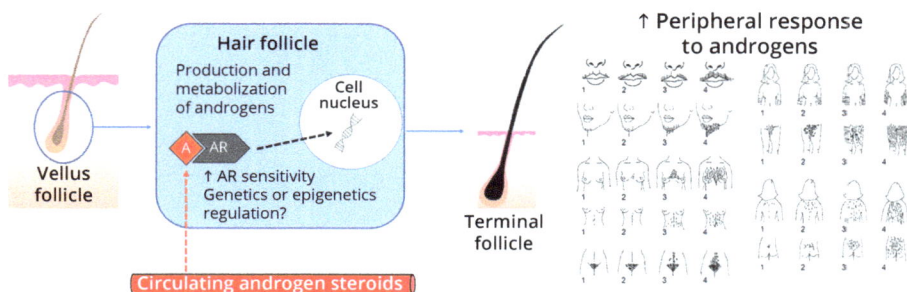

Figure I-2-1. Role of androgens in the hair follicle and its peripheral response. A — androgens; AR — androgen receptor; ↑ peripheral response to androgens is expressed graphically by the modified Ferriman–Gallwey scale (adapted from Spritzer P.M. et al., 2022)

In women with excessive androgen levels, there is a transformation of weakly-colored downy hair into thick and pigmented terminal hair on more extensive areas of the body, such as the lower abdomen, the inner surface of the thighs, the nipples and sternum, above the sacrum, and on the shoulders (**Fig. I-2-1**) (Spritzer P.M. et al., 2022). Hair growth is also observed on the face: above the upper lip, on the chin, and in the sideburn area (**Fig. I-2-2**).

Although hyperandrogenemia is found in 80–90% of women with hirsutism, the severity of hirsutism and the level of androgen excess are not always directly correlated. In idiopathic hirsutism, excessive hair growth occurs against a background of normal ovulatory function and ovarian morphology, as well as normal serum androgen levels (Unluhizarci K. et al., 2023). Presumably, in idiopathic hirsutism, the sensitivity of hair follicle receptors to androgens is increased, so even with normal levels of sex hormones, patients experience manifestations of hyperandrogenism.

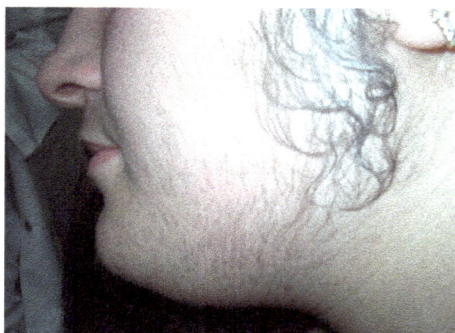

Figure I-2-2. Hirsutism depicted in a female patient with PCOS and non-classic congenital adrenal hyperplasia (adapted from Gacaferri Lumezi B. et al., 2014)

It is clear that hair removal alone cannot address the problem, and appropriate drug therapy is necessary. In a study involving 200 patients with PCOS and hirsutism after a course of complex therapy (spirono-lactone + oral contraceptives), 85% of participants observed a persistent and long-term reduction in the severity of hirsutism. The average improvement in the hirsutism severity score on the Ferriman–Gallwey scale was approximately 60% (Ezeh U. et al., 2018).

2.2. Hypertrichosis

Hypertrichosis manifests as an excessive growth of vellus and/or terminal hair in any area of the body, surpassing the normal amount for individuals of a specific age, race, and sex.

It is important to distinguish hypertrichosis from hirsutism. Hypertrichosis can occur in both women and men, while hirsutism affects only women in whom male-type terminal hair grows in androgen-dependent areas. In other words, hirsutism is a consequence of increased androgen levels and is associated with other symptoms of hyperandrogenism.

There are several classifications of hypertrichosis: by age of appearance — congenital and acquired; by the degree of spread — generalized and focal; and by the affected area — hypertrichosis of the elbows, auricles, lumbosacral spine, and other body parts.

2.2.1. Congenital hypertrichosis

Congenital generalized hypertrichosis

Congenital generalized hypertrichosis (**Fig. I-2-3**) accompanies several rare inherited syndromes in which genetic errors lead to dysfunction of

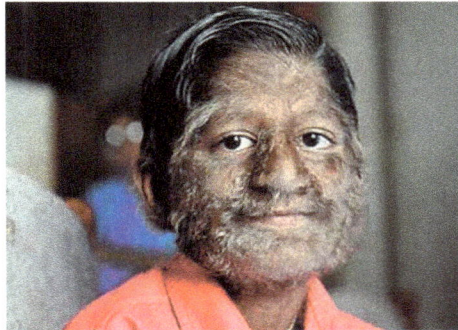

Figure I-2-3. Congenital hypertrichosis (werewolf syndrome) (photo by Ashland Science Wiki)

proteins involved in hair follicle development. The entire body of these patients is covered with long vellus hair, except in areas where hair does not usually grow (palms, feet).

There is some evidence that intrauterine exposure to drugs such as minoxidil may predispose an individual to congenital generalized hypertrichosis.

Congenital focal hypertrichosis

Congenital focal hypertrichosis is inherited in an autosomal dominant manner. Conditions belonging to this category include hairy elbow syndrome and hereditary hypertrichoses of the palms and soles, the auricle, the tip of the nose, and the anterior or posterior surface of the neck. Trichomegaly of the eyelashes is an exception, as it is an autosomal recessive disorder.

Focal hypertrichosis can occur alongside other forms of congenital pathology, including congenital melanocytic nevus, Becker's nevus, spinal dysraphism (incomplete closure of the spinal canal), and others. In the latter case, the focus of hypertrichosis is found in the lumbosacral region along the midline of the back and is commonly known as "Faun tail" (**Fig. I-2-4**). The presence of a skin abnormality along the midline of the back serves as a characteristic and reliable marker of spinal pathology: skin manifestations can occur in more than 50% of cases of spinal dysraphism (Khurana K. et al., 2023).

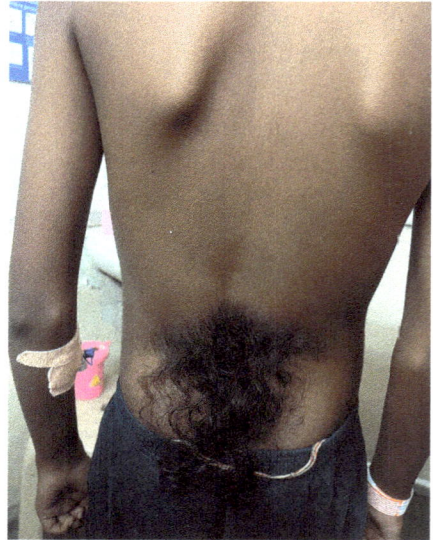

Figure I-2-4. Lumbosacral hypertrichosis ("Faun tail"), a marker of congenital spinal pathology (adapted from Khurana K. et al., 2023)

Prepubertal hypertrichosis

Prepubertal hypertrichosis is characterized by excessive growth of vellus hair on androgen-independent areas of the body during pre-pubescence. This condition is sometimes referred to as "racial hirsut-ism" due to its higher prevalence in Mediterranean and South Asian regions. Unlike true hirsutism, prepubertal hypertrichosis is not asso-ciated with androgen activity.

2.2.2. Acquired hypertrichosis

Acquired generalized hypertrichosis

Acquired generalized hypertrichosis is most often related to ad-verse side-effects of drug therapy (Elosua-González M. et al., 2018; Souza K.F. et al., 2020; Barbareschi M. et al., 2021).

The following drugs most commonly cause generalized hypertri-chosis:

- Antibiotics (streptomycin)
- Anti-inflammatory drugs (benoxaprofen, corticosteroids)
- Vasodilators (diazoxide, minoxidil, prostaglandin E1)
- Diuretics (acetazolamide)
- Anticonvulsants (phenytoin)
- Immunosuppressants (cyclosporine, mycophenolate mofetil)
- Psoralens (methoxypsoralen, trimethylpsoralen)
- Antiseptic agents (hexachlorobenzene)
- Chelators (penicillamine)
- Interferon-alpha
- Fenoterol
- Epidermal growth factor receptor inhibitors (cetuximab, panitu-mumab, erlotinib, gefitinib)

Although medications are usually the culprit, acquired generalized hypertrichosis has also been linked to traumatic brain injury, juvenile hypothyroidism, juvenile dermatomyositis, acromegaly, malnutrition, and advanced HIV infection.

Acquired hypertrichosis lanugo-type

Acquired hypertrichosis lanugo-type (or hypertrichosis lanuginosa acquisita, HLA) is often associated with metabolic and endocrine disorders, as well as the use of certain medications. The first instance of HLA in malignant tumors was recorded in 1865, and since then this syndrome has been described as a paraneoplastic syndrome in 56 patients of both sexes. HLA is sometimes found concurrently with acanthosis nigricans, papillary hypertrophy of the tongue, and glossitis. Notably, this condition is observed more frequently in women. Malignancy-associated HLA appears to be particularly common in the 40–70 age group. Among women with malignancy-associated HLA, colorectal cancer is the most prevalent, followed by lung cancer and breast cancer; in men, lung cancer is most common, followed by colorectal cancer (Slee P.H. et al., 2007).

Acquired localized hypertrichosis

Acquired localized hypertrichosis (ALH) occurs at the site of repetitive trauma, friction, irritation, or chronic inflammation. For example, ALH is often observed on the backs of sack bearers, over fractured limbs after plaster bandaging, and on the backs of the necks in weightlifters. It can also occur at vaccination sites and scars from chickenpox. In the literature, this condition has been reported at wart removal sites and after laser hair removal. ALH can also be iatrogenic: cases of hypertrichosis after psoralen plus ultraviolet-A radiation (PUVA) therapy, topical application of corticosteroids, tacrolimus, creams containing mercury or iodine, anthralin, and prostaglandin F2α analogues (latanoprost, bimatoprost) have been described (Özyurt S., Çetinkaya G.S., 2015).

Patients presenting with signs of hypertrichosis and hirsutism require a medical examination and consultation with a general practitioner, dermatologist, endocrinologist, and oncologist. Determining the cause of abnormal hair growth will clarify the prospects for the aesthetic correction of unwanted hair because, in most cases, the primary goal is to treat the underlying disease and eliminate the etiological factors that caused hirsutism or hypertrichosis.

Chapter 3
Hair features to consider when choosing a hair removal technique

Many factors influence the choice and effectiveness of hair removal techniques. An essential aspect of hair biology is the presence of a basic unit, the hair follicle, which produces the temporary structure (hair fiber). Persistent removal of unwanted hair can only be accomplished by targeting the hair follicle. This raises the question: what must be done to it to cause irreversible hair loss? Does it need to be destroyed, or is it possible to identify a specific target among the follicular structures?

The difficulty in getting rid of unwanted hair lies in the fact that HF is a very tenacious structure. It is capable of regeneration even after almost complete destruction. It is assumed that a prerequisite for regeneration is preserving the stem cells of the bulge zone. This view is confirmed by experimental data: the upper part of the follicle with the bulge zone, when transplanted to hairless mice, regenerates with the formation of a bulb and dermal papilla. From this observation, we can conclude that the target for successful permanent hair removal should most likely be HF with pluripotent bulge zone cells. It should be noted that stem cells are not only found in this zone, but their concentration is maximized there. Another target is, as we stated above, the dermal papilla, which provides nutrients to the hair follicle.

3.1. Hair types

When evaluating hair before the procedure, practitioners should consider the hair type — downy (vellus) or terminal (ostium), as well as thickness — fine, normal, or thick hair.

Recall that the vellus is fine, colorless hair that covers almost the entire body, except for those areas covered by terminal hairs. Terminal hairs are stiff, pigmented hairs on the scalp, as well as the mustache, beard, and eyebrow areas. The growth of terminal hair, as well as the process of transformation of vellus hair into terminal hair, is under the direct control of androgens. Therefore, this type of hair grows on androgen-dependent areas of the body. In normal women, these areas include the anogenital area and axillae.

Terminal hairs contain melanin and are an accessible target for light radiation. In contrast, downy hair is more resistant to removal by this technique due to the lack of melanin. Generally, facial hair is finer and lighter in color than hair on the rest of the body, making it one of the most challenging targets for light-based removal techniques. Therefore, eliminating facial hair may require a few more treatments than usual (Goel A., Rai K., 2022).

3.2. Hair growth phase

HFs are safely hidden deep within the skin and are not easy to reach without damaging the surrounding tissue. Regardless of the hair removal technique, the hair canal and hair shaft are the most direct and natural way to access the follicle. However, this pathway is not always available, but only during the active growth stage (anagen) — it is during this period of the hair's lifecycle that the hair shaft is best developed and firmly connected to the follicle. This means that the epilation outcome depends on the hair growth stage. **The most sensitive to epilation will be those HFs that are in the anagen (active growth) stage, especially in the early phase, as there is a lot of melanin in the skin at this time and the follicles are located deep in the skin and still attached to the papilla for nourishment** (Goel A., Rai K., 2022).

However, at the time of treatment, not all hair in the treated area is in the anagen stage, so it is not possible to eliminate the problem of unwanted hair in one session. According to the available data, a 20% reduction in HF number can be achieved in each session using the correct light parameters (Thomas M.M., Houreld N.N., 2019). To determine the treatment frequency, it is essential to consider that not only

Table I-2-1. Proportion of hair on different body parts in the anagen and telogen phases, duration of the telogen phase, follicle density and depth

ZONE	% OF HAIR IN THE TELOGEN PHASE	% OF HAIR IN THE ANAGEN PHASE	TELOGEN PHASE, weeks	ANAGEN PHASE, weeks	FOLLICLE DENSITY, follicles/cm^2	FOLLICLE DEPTH, mm
Head	13	85	12–16	2–6 years	350	3–5
Eyebrows	90	10	12	4–8	—	2–2.5
Ears	85	15	12	4–8	—	—
Cheeks	30–50	50–70			880	—
Beard	30	70	10	52	500	2–4
The area above the upper lip	35	65	6	16	500	1.0–2.5
Armpits	70	30	12	16	65	3.5–4.5
Pubic area	70	30	12	≥ 4	70	3.5–4.5
Hands	80	20	18	13	60	—
Thighs and shins	80	20	24	16	60	2.5–4
Mammary glands	70	30	—	—	65	3.0–4.5

the proportion of hair in the anagen and telogen phases but also the duration of the telogen phase, follicle density, and depth of follicles vary in different areas of the body (**Table I-2-1**). Additionally, the armpit and bikini areas are androgen-sensitive and should be treated about once every 1.5 months. On the face, where almost all hair is in the anagen phase, sessions are repeated every 30–45 days (initially, it is advisable to have the hair removal treatment at least once every 2 weeks), while on the arms and legs, where hair in a "dormant" state predominates, spacing sessions by 2–3 months is recommended.

The hair removal effectiveness is also influenced by gender: men have thicker epidermis, their skin produces more sebum, and follicles are located deeper. Consequently, it is more difficult to reach them.

3.3. Melanin distribution in hair and skin

Hair and skin color are paramount when it comes to light-assisted hair removal. It depends on a combination of racial, genetic, age, and endocrine factors. Caucasians can have hair of almost any color — red, blond, black, or brown. At the same time, other races may have only black or dark-brown hair.

In light-assisted hair removal, melanin is the main chromophore on which most of the light energy is focused. Therefore, a clear understanding that black, blond, red, and gray hair respond differently to the light pulse is particularly important for selecting the correct treatment parameters. However, a serious problem with light-assisted hair removal is that melanin is not only present in the hair, but also in the skin. Consequently, light energy will be absorbed not only by the hair, but also by the skin, which can lead to overheating and even burns — the darker the skin, the more likely they are to occur (see Part II, section 1.2).

The presence of a tan is another essential factor to consider when choosing a hair removal technique. Light-based treatments in patients with tanned skin can cause the epidermal melanin to absorb energy, potentially leading to burns. To reduce the likelihood of this adverse outcome, some practitioners may use suboptimal light intensity, which diminishes the procedure's effectiveness. For these reasons, the radiation wavelength should be adjusted, or an alternative hair removal technique should be chosen (Goel A., Rai K., 2022).

Hair color and thickness, as well as the patient's skin color, are indirect criteria that allow experienced practitioners to predict the therapeutic effect. For example, dark and thick hair on pale skin is the most accessible target for light-assisted hair removal. Such a clinical picture, all other things being equal, suggests a relatively quick and successful result.

Part II

Hair removal techniques

The history of combating unwanted body hair goes back thousands of years. In ancient Egypt, the first razors were invented and were used by both men and women. Shaving tools were first made of flint, then of bronze. In hot climates, shaving hair had an aesthetic and a hygienic function, as hair could become a source of odor and infection. The ancient Egyptians invented other hair removal techniques — with hot wax or resin (waxing) and with honey or sugar molasses (sugaring) — which have remained popular to this day. In Eastern countries, men did not give importance to the hair growth on the body, but women regularly used wax. Because of this prevailing practice, in Europe, this hair removal technique became known as Persian.

In ancient Greece, ladies used bronze tweezers to remove hair, as mentioned by Aristophanes in Lysistrata. Alexander the Great's warriors picked up on this strategy during their eastern campaigns and brought back a simple but very effective way of hair pulling: a coarse thread was rolled over the body, winding the hair, and then pulled sharply.

Numerous techniques for eliminating hair — both permanent and temporary — are available on the modern market. Permanent hair removal, known as **epilation**, involves the irreversible destruction of hair follicles, leading to the permanent loss of the ability to produce hair fibers. Temporary removal (**depilation**) involves the removal of the outer part of the hair — the shaft — which may or may not cause reversible damage to the hair follicle.

Epilation involves not just removing the hair shaft but also destroying the hair follicle (HF) so that the hair can no longer grow. The HF is the main target of all epilation techniques; however, because it is located deep beneath the skin's surface, reaching it without damaging the underlying layers is challenging. Among the modern hair removal techniques, the following stand out:

1. Light-assisted hair removal
2. Electrical hair removal
3. Ultrasound-assisted hair removal
4. Enzyme-based hair removal

Common contraindications to hair removal include:
- Skin diseases in the stage of exacerbation
- Pregnancy
- Varicose veins (at the site of the procedure)
- Skin malignancies
- Infectious diseases
- Tendency to form keloid scars
- Clotting disorder
- Violation of skin integrity (wounds, abrasions, lacerations, cuts, crusts)
- Active herpes
- Diabetes
- Hypertension
- Ischemic heart disease
- Epilepsy

Unlike epilation, depilation has a short-lived effect because only the outer part of the hair shaft is removed, while the source of the hair — the hair follicle — remains intact or suffers minimal damage. Most depilation treatments are simple, quick, and inexpensive, and many can be easily used at home.

Depilation techniques include:
- Shaving
- Plucking or pulling (using tweezers, thread)
- Chemical depilation with the help of special cosmetic products
- Waxing, sugaring

Chapter 1
Light-assisted hair removal

Light-assisted epilation, which uses light energy to destroy the HF, is currently considered the most promising. It is based on the mechanism of selective photothermolysis.

1.1. Mechanism of action

The theory of selective photothermolysis was formulated by Richard Anderson and John Parrish of the Wellman Center for Photomedicine at Harvard Medical School. Their idea was grounded in the point effect of a laser beam on the substance — the chromophore, the concentration of which in the target cell is much higher than in the neighboring cells. The light parameters (wavelength, intensity, and duration of irradiation) are selected in accordance with the absorption spectrum of the chromophore as the aim is to transfer as much energy as possible to its molecules. After absorbing quanta of light, the chromophore enters an excited state, while the reverse transition is accompanied by the release of "excess" energy into the surrounding space in the form of heat. Thus, under the action of light, heating occurs, causing irreversible destruction of both the target cell and (if necessary) its nearest neighbors (**enhanced selective photothermolysis**).

In the case of light-assisted hair removal, the main biological targets are the cells responsible for hair growth: the mature keratinocytes that directly produce hair (located in the dermal papilla) and stem cells (located in the bulge area and in the niche above the dermal papilla). Unfortunately, neither of these has a chromophore that can be selectively acted upon by light energy. However, an appropriate chromophore is present in melanocytes located among keratinocytes in the lower part of the hair follicle, as well as in keratinized hair shaft cells filled with melanin.

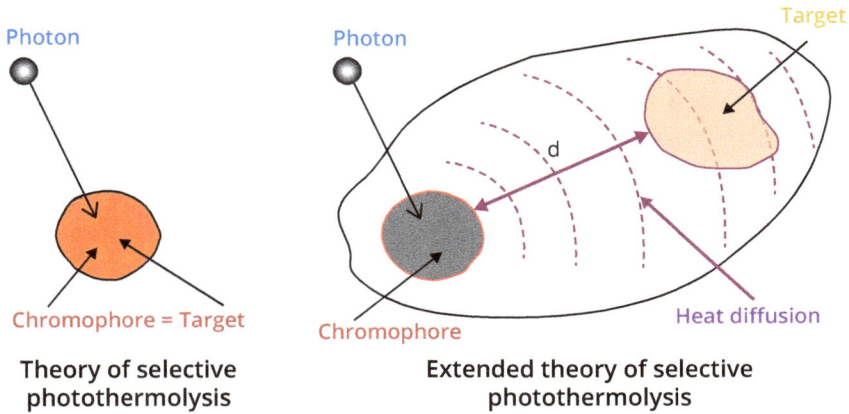

Figure II-1-1. Selective photothermolysis vs. extended selective photothermolysis

Melanin is the chromophore for light-assisted hair removal. It absorbs light in the red and infrared (IR) regions very well, after which it becomes excited. As such excited state cannot be maintained, it returns to its normal state by giving off energy in the form of heat, which damages primarily the melanocytes and nearby living cells. Thus, the melanocytes of the hair follicle are the generators of heat that destroys the target keratinocytes of the hair follicle, stem cells, and the dermal papilla (**Fig. II-1-1**).

Proceeding from the above, in the case of light-assisted hair removal, it would be more correct to speak about the effects postulated by the theory of **extended selective photothermolysis**, according to which the secondary heat has a pronounced effect on the target, which may be located at some distance from the heat generator (Altshuler G.B. et al., 2001).

This poses a dilemma for the engineers designing the hair removal devices and the operators who conduct light-assisted hair removal procedures regarding the optimal radiation parameters to achieve the desired thermal effect:

1. On the one hand, the delivered light energy must be **sufficient** not just to overcome the distance between melanocytes and stem cells, but to thermally destroy the latter.
2. On the other hand, it needs to be **insufficient** for causing damage to the interfollicular epidermis and adjacent dermis.

In fact, the entire evolution of light-based hair removal technologies reflects the search for a solution to this issue, which most directly relates to the procedure efficacy/safety aspects and client tolerance.

HFs in the phase of active growth (anagen) are the most sensitive to damage. Prominent pigmentation and active growth are the keys to their successful photothermal destruction.

The effect of light-assisted hair removal is progressive: hair growth continues to slow down, and the number of hairs decreases after the course of epilation is completed. While the exact mechanism of hair growth impairment during light-assisted hair removal remains unknown, several mechanisms are apparently involved (Ibrahimi O.A. et al., 2011).

1. Heat exposure causes the vessels that supply the hair follicle to coagulate, leading to gradual atrophy of the follicle and cessation of hair growth.
2. Heat exposure triggers programmed death in the cells of the follicular epithelium, leading to follicular atrophy.
3. The regulation of growth phases is disrupted due to the disarrangement of interactions between the follicle growth cells.

1.2. Hair and skin features to be considered during light-assisted hair removal

Melanin, the target chromophore in light-assisted hair removal, is found in both hair and skin. We need to damage the melanin in the hair but not the melanin in the epidermis, so the color of the hair and skin is particularly important.

Color depends on many factors, the most important of which are genetic and endocrine. As we have already said, a wide range of hair color — from the lightest to jet-black — is formed mainly by two pigments: black–brown eumelanin and yellow–red pheomelanin, which differ in the granule size. Variants depend on the quantitative ratio of these pigments, while the change in hair color during life is due to the dynamics of the general endocrine background. Both eumelanin and pheomelanin are synthesized in melanocytes located in the hair follicle above the papilla. Melanocytes produce pigment only during the growth stage. To determine the correct principles of light-assisted hair removal, it is important to understand that black, blond, red, and gray hair may respond differently to the light pulse.

But melanin (eumelanin and pheomelanin) is also present in the skin. Different people's skin varies in its ability to produce melanin, the distribution of melanocytes, and its blood supply. The lighter the skin and the less melanin it contains, the less "competitive" its absorption of laser energy. At the same time, individuals with darker skin phototypes have an excess of melanin. The same issue arises in people with a tan. Due to the high melanin content, the skin can become very hot and may even burn during light-assisted hair removal, while hair follicles and hair shafts "under-receive" the required amount of radiation and are not completely destroyed. As a result, dark-skinned patients experience a higher incidence of adverse reactions to light-assisted hair removal than light-skinned patients. Specialists attempt to overcome this limitation by experimenting with different wavelengths, energy densities, and other parameters.

Thomas Fitzpatrick developed a classification of skin types based on the skin's ability to respond to ultraviolet (UV) radiation (**Table II-1-1**). The same classification is used to predict the outcome of light-assisted hair removal and to select the radiation source.

Table II-1-1. Skin phototypes according to Fitzpatrick

PHOTOTYPE	CHARACTERIZATION	HAIR COLOR
I	Never tans, always burns (milky-white skin, blue/green eyes)	Light-colored or red
II	Can sometimes tan, but more often burns (fair skin, green/brown eyes)	Blond or brown
III	Often tans, sometimes burns (golden skin, brown eyes)	Chestnut
IV	Always tans, never burns (olive skin, dark eyes)	Black or dark brown
V	Never burns (dark-brown skin, black eyes)	Black
VI	Black	Black

Nowadays, light-assisted hair removal can be performed on people with any skin and hair color, but it is crucial to choose the proper radiation parameters. However, patients with black and brown hair, on average, achieve better results than those with red or blond hair. In addition, the longer the radiation wavelength, the less effective epilation will be in the latter group, because long-wavelength radiation is poorly absorbed by melanin, which is already scarce in light-colored hair. In general, it can be said that epilation of light hair is less effective than dark hair. Patients with light hair can usually achieve a temporary reduction in the number of hairs for up to 12 weeks, while most patients with brown and black hair have a delay in growth of 2 to 6 months after one session.

The skin on different parts of the body also differs in the thickness of the epidermis and the depth of hair (**Fig. II-1-2**). There are also gender differences — men tend to have thicker epidermis, more fat-producing skin, and deeper follicles.

A good response to light-assisted hair removal occurs when the target hair has a high concentration of chromophores. Accordingly, terminal (long, dense) hairs are the best candidates for this procedure.

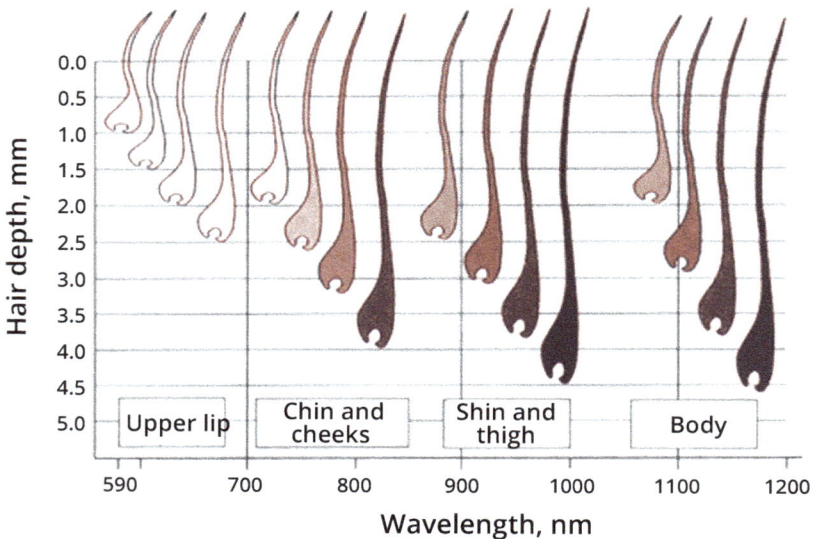

Figure II-1-2. Selection of the radiation wavelength depending on the hair color, location, and depth

Conversely, vellus (short, light-colored) hairs contain little melanin and consequently absorb light energy poorly, making them difficult to destroy. This statement holds true when treating areas such as that above the upper lip, where the chromophore is present in lower amounts, but the hair itself is quite thin. In general, regarding size, epilation of hair with a diameter below 30 μm is not particularly effective.

1.3 Light-assisted hair removal devices

Depending on the light source, two epilation techniques are distinguished:
1. **Laser hair removal** — exposure to monochromatic light from a laser source
2. **IPL hair removal** — exposure to intense flashes of broadband light generated by a flash lamp

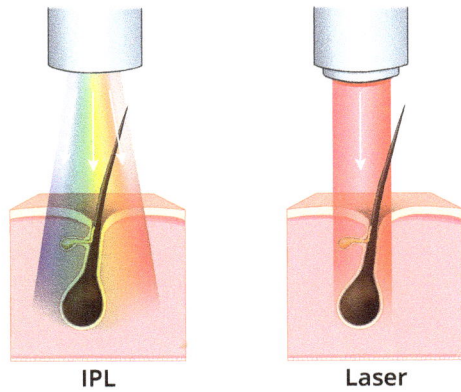

IPL   Laser

Figure II-1-3. Schematic representation of the differences between IPL and laser radiation (image by Wikipedia)

Both variants of light-assisted hair removal have been used successfully, but there are some notable differences between them (**Fig. II-1-3**).

1.3.1. Laser devices

Lasers can create a radiation stream that has unique properties of monochromaticity, coherence, and collimation.

Monochromaticity. All electromagnetic waves emitted by the laser have one wavelength (λ); for example, the ruby laser — λ = 694 nm, and the erbium laser (Er:YAG) — λ = 2940 nm. Due to the high degree of monochromaticity, laser radiation exhibits a high **spectral density**, meaning there is an increased concentration of light energy at one wavelength. This provides the necessary exposure power and ensures accuracy in targeting the absorption peak of the target chromophore.

Coherence. Lasers generate electromagnetic oscillations that are synchronized in phase — the waves propagate as if "in time." This ensures maximal laser focus.

Collimation. Laser radiation forms a parallel beam of light that does not scatter with distance. This characteristic allows for high brightness and maximizes the percentage of delivered energy that can be focused on the target.

1.3.2. IPL devices

IPL (intense pulsed light) devices generate broadband pulsed light, meaning they emit radiation at various wavelengths. As a result, IPL devices are characterized by what is known as **polychromatic radiation**, with wavelengths ranging from 400 to 1200 nm, which correspond to the visible and near-IR parts of the spectrum. By using light filters, it is possible to select the required wavelength for a specific procedure or to utilize the entire available range.

The second feature of IPL technology is **incoherence**. This means that the electromagnetic waves emitted by the lamp do not coincide with each other in phase, but rather oscillate uncoordinated (i.e., apart), which broadens the beam focus.

Finally, the third specific feature of IPL is its **non-collimated** nature. Unlike lasers, which are characterized by narrow directionality, IPL devices generate divergent beams of light. This slightly reduces the intensity of their impact but expands the irradiation zone — a much larger area is treated in one flash.

The ability of IPL devices to generate a wide range of wavelengths absorbed by different skin chromophores is both an advantage and a disadvantage. On the one hand, IPL technology enables several major chromophores to be affected simultaneously, allowing practitioners to address many aesthetic problems with a single device. On the other hand, the energy of the emitted light is distributed among all these chromophores, primarily affecting the superficial layers while deeper targets receive less energy.

In the case of hair removal, this problem is less of an issue than when addressing other aesthetic concerns, because the hair shaft itself serves as a light guide due to its increased melanin content, directing the energy to the HF. However, the large spot size is certainly a concern; while it enables faster treatment, it limits the application of laser-like energy levels due to the risk of damaging non-target tissues. Consequently, IPL epilation is generally regarded as less effective than laser hair removal, although modern devices facilitate very effective treatments.

1.4. Light exposure parameters

The following basic conditions must be met to realize high exposure selectivity:

- **Optical selectivity** — the chromophore of the target structure should have a higher absorption coefficient for radiation of a given wavelength than chromophores in the surrounding tissues.
- **Thermal selectivity** — the exposure time should be equal to or lower than the thermal relaxation time (TRT) of the target structure (TRT is the period required to transfer 63% of the received heat — reduction of thermal energy equal to e = 2.7 times — to the surrounding tissues), so that the energy imparted by the light pulse to the biological object is used only for its heating and destruction, but is not transferred to the surrounding tissues. However, in the case of epilation, the exposure time must be greater than the TRT of melanin, because the light-assisted hair removal principle is based on the concept of enhanced selective photothermolysis — **the energy must be transferred beyond the structures containing the target chromophores**. Thus, while the TRT of melanosomes is 250 ns, the TRT of hair follicles is 10–100 ms.
- **Energy selectivity** — **sufficient energy** is needed to destroy the target.

All these conditions can be met by selecting the exposure parameters of both laser and IPL systems. The main parameters affecting the effectiveness and safety of light-assisted hair removal treatment are:

- Radiation wavelength (nm)
- Energy flux density (fluence) (J/cm^2)
- Light spot size (mm)
- Pulse duration (ms)
- Protecting the epidermis from burns

1.4.1. Wavelength

When choosing a wavelength of radiation for hair removal, we are guided by the concept known as the **melanin window**, which reflects the spectral range in which it makes sense to work if we want to affect melanin and minimize the impact on other chromophores (**Table II-1-2**). The melanin window includes radiation generated by ruby (694 nm), alexandrite (755 nm), diode (800–810 nm), and neodymium-doped yttrium aluminum garnet / Nd:YAG (1064 nm) lasers, as well as non-laser IPL devices (intense pulsed light over a wide range, 400–1200 nm, with the specific spectrum controlled by filters). All of these light sources, except the ruby laser, are currently used in specific light-assisted hair removal devices, indicating that there is no "best" light source.

Table II-1-2. Absorption coefficients of major skin chromophores as a function of wavelength

LIGHT RADIATION								
Wavelength, nm	410	532	595	694	755	810	940	1064
Depth of light penetration into the skin, μm	100	350	550	750	1000	1200	1500	1700
CHROMOPHORE	ABSORPTION COEFFICIENT, cm^{-1}							
Oxyhemoglobin	2000	190	35	1.2	2.3	3.6	5.2	2.2
Deoxyhemoglobin	1300	140	96	6.6	5.2	2.7	3.0	0.6
Melanin	140	56	38	23	17	13	7	5.7
Water	6.7×10^{-5}	4.4×10^{-4}	1.7×10^{-3}	5.9×10^{-3}	0.029	0.022	0.18	0.144

There is an important problem to note: since melanin is also contained in the skin, radiation that is very well absorbed by it will be dangerous for the skin of dark phototypes. Therefore, although the alexandrite laser provides effective hair removal, it can only be used on light skin (phototypes I–III). The greater the contrast between the degree of hair and skin pigmentation, the safer the light-assisted hair removal. Therefore, for people with dark phototypes, lasers that generate radiation that is less actively absorbed by melanin — diode (800–810 nm) and Nd:YAG (1064 nm) — should be used. Diode lasers are the most universal and can be used to treat skin of any phototype. The specifics of the Nd:YAG mechanism of action will be discussed below.

While the radiation wavelength is fixed, modern devices for light-assisted hair removal allow for adjustments to the density of energy flow, pulse duration, and sometimes even the size of the light spot in accordance with the skin phototype and patient characteristics (in particular, the threshold of sensitivity).

1.4.2. Fluence and light spot size

Energy density (fluence) is the main variable parameter of exposure, which determines the procedure effectiveness. Its value indicates how much light energy (J) is transmitted per unit of skin surface (cm^2). Thus, the energy received by the HF depends on the **pulse energy** and **spot size**.

For example, 100 J distributed across a surface measuring 1 × 1 cm^2 (1 cm^2) corresponds to an energy density of 100 J/cm^2. If delivered to a 2 × 2 cm^2 (i.e., 4 cm^2) area, the energy density is reduced to 25 J/cm^2. The higher the energy density, the more energy is transferred to the hair shaft and HF. Conversely, if the spot size is large, a greater number of follicles can be affected in one flash.

The size of the light spot also determines another important parameter — the adequate depth of exposure. The skin scatters light, limiting the delivery of the necessary energy to deep-lying chromophores, which is crucial in the case of epilation or removal of vascular defects. Increasing the light spot size can reduce energy loss due to scattering and allow more photons to reach the target.

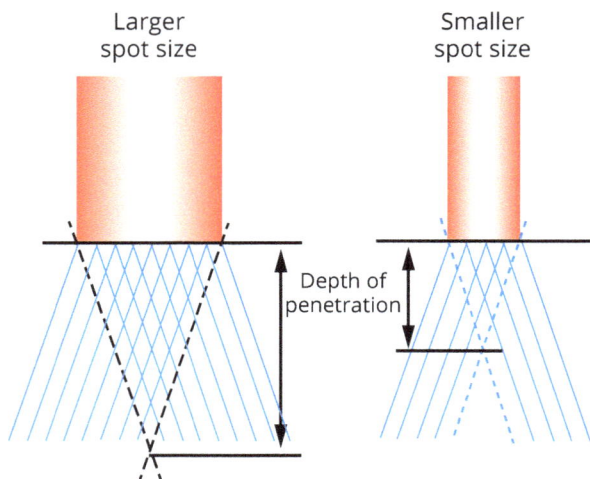

Larger spot size

Smaller spot size

Depth of penetration

Figure II-1-4.
Dependence of the radiation penetration depth on the laser spot size

If a more superficial effect is desired, the spot size should be reduced (**Fig. II-1-4**).

1.4.3. Pulse duration

Thermal energy is delivered to the HF indirectly — through the conductor (hair shaft), and thus requires more time. For this reason, long-pulsed lasers operating in the 10–100 ms range or even higher are used for epilation.

At the same time, a pulse that is too long is dangerous, as it would transfer excessive heat to the surrounding tissues and cause thermal damage. This problem can be addressed by using devices that generate a series of sub-pulses with short inter-pulse intervals, allowing the epidermis and dermis to cool down while the hair shaft remains unaffected. Another option is to increase the radiation power and shorten the pulse duration, which will reduce the area of boundary heating and thus prevent burns to the adjacent skin.

In general, the risk of burns is much lower with IPL devices, as the flashes of light are separated by quite long intervals and the skin has time to cool down.

1.4.4. Protecting the epidermis from burns

To protect the epidermis when using laser systems, modern laser hair removal devices utilize three cooling options:
- Contact: a cold plate (glass, sapphire, or metal) is located on the working arm of the device
- Air: cold air is emitted from the device
- Dynamic: using cryogenic spray

Contact cooling is considered the most effective. It should be noted that the skin should be cooled not only during the procedure, but also before and after it. If this is done, epilation is easier to tolerate and swelling and pain sensations are less pronounced.

However, the risk of burns cannot be eliminated entirely. The risk increases in the following cases:
- When the skin surrounding the follicle has high melanin content
- When both hair density and hair shaft thickness are high
- When high pulse energy and radiation power is used
- When long pulses are delivered

In each specific case, the radiation energy and pulse duration must be selected based on the characteristics of the patient's skin and hair. At the same time, the success of epilation is completely determined by the choice of the radiation source, its technical characteristics, its mode of operation, and the cooling systems utilized.

1.5. Devices for light-assisted hair removal

1.5.1. Long-pulsed lasers

A high-density laser beam can produce a significant local thermal effect, which is accompanied by coagulation of the follicular zone, vaporization (dehydration), and carbonization (charring) of the tissue surrounding the follicle. In other words, the follicle is burned, dried, and charred. The special software of the laser systems allows

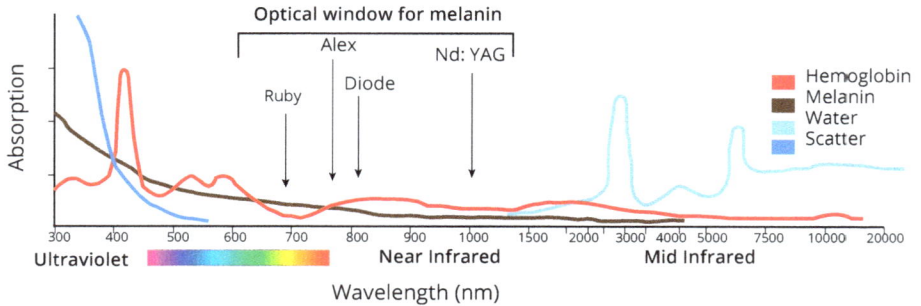

Figure II-1-5. Absorption spectra of skin chromophores

for precisely targeted selective action, so that all these effects take place only in the HF area.

In addition to thermal effects, light produces other effects (photo-electric, biostimulating, etc.), but thermal effects predominate when the power of the radiation source is high.

Destruction of the hair follicle with a laser beam is possible only if there is a chromophore in the path of the beam that absorbs radiation in the red part of the spectrum (radiation of this wavelength penetrates the skin the deepest) and is concentrated mainly in the hair, otherwise the beam is spontaneously deactivated (it is scattered). This natural chromophore is melanin, which is present in high quantities in the hair shaft.

Based on the absorption spectrum of melanin and other skin chromophores, ruby, alexandrite, diode, and Nd:YAG lasers provide the most suitable radiation for epilation (**Fig. II-1-5**).

Ruby laser

The ruby laser was the first to appear on the laser hair removal market. It generates red radiation with a wavelength of 694 nm, producing light pulses of about 3 ms duration and providing an energy flow of up to 40–60 J/cm². The pulse repetition rate is 1 Hz, meaning it is a relatively slow-acting laser. Since the target here is exclusively the melanin of the hair follicle (hemoglobin absorbs weakly at this wavelength), ruby laser cannot be used on tanned skin because its energy will be dissipated, and there is a high risk of damage to soft tissue. In addition, it does not "recognize" light-colored hair.

Ruby laser epilation produces the best results when removing dark hair from light skin. Blond and red hair, as well as hair on tanned skin and on skin phototypes IV and V, remain largely unaffected. However, sometimes ruby laser treatment does not yield the desired effect even on dark hair. Interestingly, after treatment, the follicle typically does not die but instead enters the catagen and then the telogen phase. The cessation of hair growth is achieved by disrupting the growth cycle.

Alexandrite laser

Alexandrite laser generates radiation with a wavelength of 755 nm, which coincides with minimal absorption by hemoglobin and strong absorption by melanin. Treatment is performed with the following parameters: spot size 10–14 mm, pulse duration 15–30 ms, pulse repetition rate 5 Hz (i.e., it is 5 times faster than ruby laser), pulse energy density 10–20 J/cm^2.

More than 95% of alexandrite laser radiation is absorbed by melanin. The absorbed energy transforms into heat, causing "burning" of the hair shaft and thermal destruction of the hair follicle and the vessels that supply it. If the hair is in the anagen phase, when there is a close connection between the vessels and the growth zone, no hair growth is observed after the procedure. Within two weeks after the procedure, there is a loss of coagulated hair "roots." Depending on the area, subsequent procedures are performed every 4–8 weeks. With each procedure, the number of hairs in the treated area decreases, and their growth rate slows down. To achieve a permanent effect of hair removal, a minimum of 5 procedures is needed, after which the treatment should be repeated 2–3 times a year to eliminate any remaining hairs.

Due to the competitive absorption of this radiation by the melanin in the interfollicular epidermis, the procedure can only be performed on skin phototypes I–IV and requires mandatory cooling to prevent burns and dyschromia. Alexandrite laser is still considered the "gold standard" for the removal of dark hair on light skin.

Neodymium laser

Hair removal with a neodymium (Nd:YAG) laser relies on the homogeneous absorption of light by oxy- and deoxyhemoglobin, as well as various protein structures, which heat up and lead to the coagulation of blood vessels and the destruction of highly differentiated cells and the germinative zones of the hair follicle. Melanin's low absorption capacity for laser energy at this wavelength (approximately 10%) eliminates competition between skin and hair pigments. Consequently, the neodymium laser does not damage the hair shaft when treating light hair, and the likelihood of experiencing complications such as dyschromia is considerably lower compared to the alexandrite laser (**Table II-1-3**).

Table II-1-3. Comparative characteristics of alexandrite and Nd:YAG laser hair removal

ALEXANDRITE LASER (755 nm)	ND:YAG (1064 nm)
"Gold standard" of dark hair removal for I–III skin phototypes	"Gold standard" hair removal for III–IV skin phototypes
Minimum course — 5 sessions	Minimum course — 8 sessions
Ineffective for light-colored hair	Effective for the removal of hair with low melanin content
Destroys melanin in the skin	Weakly absorbed by the melanin in the skin
Penetrates to a depth of about 3 mm, which is sometimes not enough	Penetrates to the entire depth of the dermis, destroys deep follicles
Painless treatment	The treatment is more painful than alexandrite hair removal

Today, Nd:YAG is regarded as the device of choice for dark skin phototypes and light hair. Due to the uniform absorption of radiation at 1064 nm by tissues, the procedure tends to be more painful than when using the alexandrite laser, making it unsuitable for all patients. The effectiveness of hair removal with this type of laser is relatively low: after a single session, 40% of hair regrows after one month, and this percentage doubles after three months. Consequently, particularly when treating light-colored hair, the amount of hair decreases only after the third session. Thus, at least eight treatments are required to achieve noticeable results.

Diode laser

Diode laser is a relatively new device belonging to the semiconductor laser category. The active medium consists of diode plates made of diode materials (based on potassium, indium, and aluminum compounds).

Diode laser generates radiation with a wavelength of 800–810 nm, belonging to the near-IR part of the spectrum, corresponding to the absorption region of not only melanin but also hemoglobin. Pulse duration ranges from 5 to 30 ms, frequency is set to 1 Hz, and energy flux on tissues is 10–40 J/cm^2 in a laser spot with a diameter of 9 mm.

The diode laser, like the ruby laser, cannot provide effective hair removal for blond and red hair, or hair on tanned skin. However, there are interesting modifications to diode lasers that partially circumvent these problems. For example, LightSheer DUET (Lumenis) combines laser radiation with vacuum action. The applicator is dome-shaped and is connected to a vacuum pump, which, when switched on, creates negative pressure, lifting the skin toward the radiating elements (**Fig. II-1-6**). Due to this effect:

- The distance between the follicles and the transmitter is reduced.
- The epidermis is stretched — the density of melanin in it decreases, and the skin adjacent to the follicle is heated to a lesser extent, decreasing the risk of thermal damage to it.

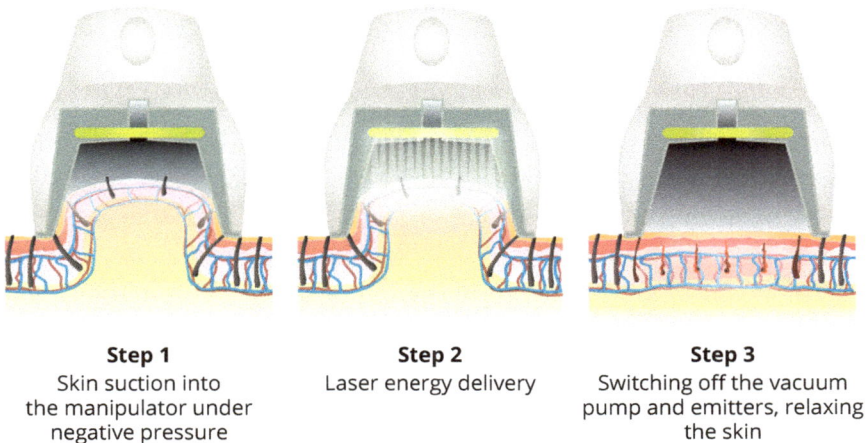

Step 1	Step 2	Step 3
Skin suction into the manipulator under negative pressure	Laser energy delivery	Switching off the vacuum pump and emitters, relaxing the skin

Figure II-1-6. Vacuum-assisted laser hair removal technology (LightSheer DUET, Lumenis)

- Partial constriction of blood vessels occurs — hemoglobin concentration in the affected area decreases.
- Light scattering is reduced due to the larger spot size and the presence of reflective surfaces (the inner "dome" surface is covered by a special coating).
- Pain sensations are reduced — due to the distracting effect of negative pressure on tactile receptors, the neurosynaptic "switch" in the spinal cord that transmits the pain impulse to the brain is blocked (according to the gate control theory of pain*) (Ibrahimi O.A., Kilmer S.L., 2012).

Thus, in the skin area located under the "dome," when the vacuum pump is switched on, there is a significant decrease in the number of competitive chromophores due to a decrease in melanin density and hemoglobin concentration. This fact, combined with the proximity of follicles to the transmitter, allows the energy flow to be reduced to about 12 J/cm^2 instead of the usual 30–40 J/cm^2, which ensures a high level of safety and provides high efficiency (hair is removed permanently after 3–4 procedures). At the same time, the spot size is large enough to conveniently treat large areas of the body. All this means that less time is required for the procedure (on average, treatment time is reduced by 60%). Local reduction of pain sensitivity makes the procedure comfortable and easily tolerated without the use of local anesthesia, although skin cooling before and after exposure is still necessary.

ELOS technology (Syneron) is also noteworthy in this context. ELOS stands for Electro-Optical Synergy — a technique that combines selective photothermolysis and tissue heating through the use of variable high-frequency radiofrequency (RF) current. This bipolar technology was originally developed to enable epilation for people with darker skin phototypes, helping to avoid burns and other complications. This

---

* The gate control theory of pain describes how non-painful sensations can override and reduce painful sensations. A painful, nociceptive stimulus stimulates primary afferent fibers and travels to the brain via transmission cells. Enhanced activity of the transmission cells results in greater perceived pain. Conversely, their suppressed activity reduces perceived pain. In the gate control theory, a closed "gate" describes blocked input to transmission cells, reducing the sensation of pain. An open "gate" permits input to transmission cells, allowing pain to be felt. — Wikipedia

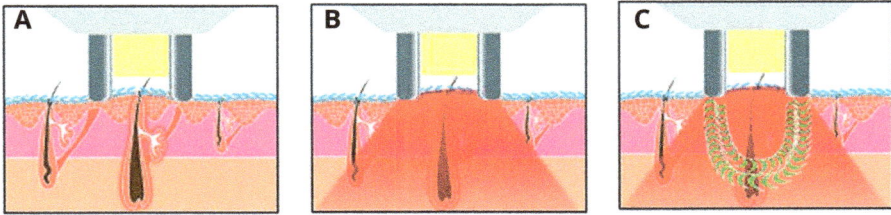

Figure II-1-7. Principle of ELOS-epilation

aim was achieved by using relatively low levels of energy, both light and electrical, with overlapping effects, through which the desired result is attained via synergy (Sadick N.S., 2005).

The ELOS effect occurs in two stages. First, the device generates light energy (diode lasers or flash lamps are used as a light source) at relatively low levels to avoid destruction while heating the tissues that contain melanin and are adjacent to them. Tissue heating is known to reduce electrical resistance, facilitating the passage of electric current. However, at the boundary with areas where resistance remains high (in this case, the hair shaft tissue), the current encounters an obstacle, and electrical energy is "concentrated" as it is converted through ion motion and dipole rotation into thermal energy (**Fig. II-1-7**). Thus, passing an electric current through laser-preheated tissue allows the cells of the matrix, dermal papilla, and bulge zone located at this boundary to heat to the coagulation temperature while keeping the remaining parts of the tissue intact. There are also devices for ELOS-epilation at home, such as Iluminage Beauty and Elos Me. Their features are similar to those of lasers and IPL devices for at-home use.

Combined laser technologies

There are devices on the market that combine several types of lasers at once, which opens up additional opportunities for specialists to select the optimal treatment parameters.

The MIX technology presented in the Duetto laser system (Quanta Systems) combines alexandrite (755 nm) and Nd:YAG (1064 nm) lasers, which allows the energy density of laser radiation to be reduced compared to monotechnology, making the procedure safer. During epilation, both types of radiation are delivered simultaneously. The 755-nm radiation is absorbed by the melanin in the hair. The melanin heats up and coagulates, and the heat spreads to the HF growth zone, but does not destroy it as the energy delivered is insufficient. However, the heating makes this zone more susceptible to the action of 1064-nm radiation, which selectively heats it to a critical temperature, leading to destruction. Thus, Nd:YAG targets the tissues "marked" by the alexandrite laser.

The new generation of diode lasers for hair removal is represented by hybrid technologies that utilize various light waves in different combinations to generate a single light pulse (**Table II-1-4**). This allows practitioners to optimize exposure parameters while considering skin phototype and hair color, thereby minimizing associated risks. The 755/810 nm configuration is suitable for working with any skin phototype and light hair, whereas the 810/1064 nm combination facilitates treatment of follicles located at varying depths to remove both light and dark hair. Most hybrid

Table II-1-4. Hybrid laser technologies vs. monochrome technologies

ALEXANDRITE, 755 nm "GOLD STANDARD" FOR DARK HAIR REMOVAL ON LIGHT SKIN (PHOTOTYPES I–II)	HYBRID DIODE, 755 nm/810 nm
The primary target is melanin	The primary target is melanin
Cannot be used in phototypes above IV due to the risk of burning the perifollicular epidermis	Can be adapted to work with any phototypes
Ineffective for light-colored hair	Removes light and fine hair
Penetrates up to 3 mm deep, which is sometimes not enough	Deeper penetration into the skin
Nd:YAG, 1064 nm "GOLD STANDARD" HAIR REMOVAL FOR SKIN PHOTOTYPES III–IV	HYBRID DIODE, 810 nm/1064 nm
The primary target is oxyhemoglobin	The main targets are melanin and oxyhemoglobin
Effective for epilation of light-colored hair with low melanin content. Poorly removes dark hair	Removes both dark and light-colored hair
Penetrates to the entire depth of the dermis, destroys deep follicles	Destroys both deep and superficial follicles
Painful treatment	Less painful treatment

hair removal lasers feature two arms based on the combination of laser diodes. More recently, devices with a single arm housing three types of diodes have emerged, combining radiation at 755, 810, and 1064 nm wavelengths (Raj Kirit E.P. et al., 2021; Gold M.H. et al., 2023).

1.5.2. Short-pulsed lasers

The lasers mentioned above are long-pulsed lasers, and their action is realized due to the photothermal effect. Short-pulsed lasers that are built on the Q-Switched (QSw)* principles are based mainly on photoacoustic (photomechanical) tissue destruction.

This mechanism is realized when a very large amount of energy is transferred to the chromophore over a very short time interval (of nano- and picosecond duration). The photoacoustic effect consists of the appearance of sound oscillations in the medium upon absorption of pulsed light and is associated with the emergence of pressure waves during the transformation of light energy into heat. It is believed that this leads to the formation of cavitation bubbles (0.1–0.2 mm in diameter) without residual thermal damage. **The shorter the pulse, the less the photothermal mechanism contributes to the target destruction and the more pronounced the photomechanical effect.**

When ultrashort high-energy pulses are absorbed by the melanin in hair, acoustic shock blast waves are formed, which cause mechanical destruction of the hair. However, it is one thing to destroy the hair shaft, and another to deliver the right amount of energy to the depth of the hair papilla without causing damage to the surrounding structures, which is much more difficult.

To solve this problem, a technology implemented in the Multiline platform (Linline GmbH) is proposed. It is based on the application of packets of nanosecond pulses with a wavelength of 1079 nm,

---

* Q-Switching technology enables a laser to produce a pulsed output beam. This technique facilitates the creation of light pulses with extremely high (gigawatt) peak power, significantly greater than what the same laser would produce if operating in continuous wave (constant output) mode. Compared to mode locking, which is another method for pulse generation with lasers, Q-switching results in much lower pulse repetition rates, much higher pulse energies, and much longer pulse durations. The two techniques can sometimes be applied simultaneously.

typically using a neodymium-doped yttrium aluminum perovskite laser (Nd:YAP) in QSw mode. This approach makes it possible to form a layer of air cavities at the boundary between the cortex and the hair cuticle. This layer serves as a heat-insulating shell that prevents heat from spreading to the adjacent skin and keeps it contained within the hair shaft. The only way for heat to disperse is downward toward the HF, resulting in thermal damage to the dermal papilla, which destroys the HF. The developers claim that this principle of action, which protects the tissues surrounding the hair, allows for the procedures to be performed on skin of different phototypes with various hair colors. Additionally, due to the less pronounced photothermal effect, no anesthesia or cooling is needed.

1.5.3. IPL

Non-monochromatic light — sourced from a long-pulsed broadband xenon lamp — can be used for hair removal. Light pulses are generated across a wide spectral range, from 500 to 1200 nm, which overlaps with the area of strong absorption by melanin. To work with pigmented structures, practitioners use filters that eliminate unnecessary radiation wavelengths, retaining only those within the "melanin window."

In contrast to lasers, the lamp projects a rectangle of up to 4.5 cm² onto the skin, allowing many more hairs to be treated in one flash. A light flux of 35–55 J/cm² is delivered by a series of up to five consecutive pulses, each ranging from 2 to 5 ms in duration. The pulses cause photothermal death of the follicle, while the intervals between pulses allow the skin to cool down.

More detailed information on light-emitting devices is available in our *Lasers in Cosmetic Dermatology & Skincare Practice* book.

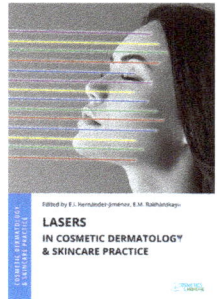

Edited by E.L. Hernández-Jiménez, E.M. Rakhmatulin

LASERS
IN COSMETIC DERMATOLOGY
& SKINCARE PRACTICE

1.6. Effectiveness of light-assisted hair removal

1.6.1. Comparative effectiveness of light-assisted hair removal devices

Laser and IPL devices provide long-lasting hair removal, but there is limited evidence regarding their long-term efficacy. This was confirmed by a systematic review of five randomized controlled trials with a follow-up period equivalent to one complete hair growth cycle for the respective body site conducted by Krasniqi A. et al. (2022). They aimed to evaluate the long-term efficacy of different light-assisted hair removal devices, considering variations in body regions that influence hair growth cycles. Based on a total sample of 223 patients, the mean long-term hair reduction with Nd:YAG ranged from 30% to 73.61%; with the alexandrite laser, it ranged from 35% to 84.25%; and with the diode laser, from 32.5% to 69.2%. For all three laser types, the most significant long-term reduction was noted for leg hair removal (with a growth cycle of 12 months), while it was the lowest for facial hair removal (6-month growth cycle). IPL provided an average long-term hair reduction of 27–52.7%, with the lowest reduction observed in the facial area and the highest in the axillary area (7-month growth cycle). The authors concluded that the **most prolonged hair reduction occurred in body areas with longer growth cycles**.

As a part of their study, Sari I.W. et al. (2023) compared the success rate of lower-extremity hair removal using IPL, alexandrite, and Nd:YAG devices. The authors analyzed the data of one male and one female patient, both aged 28 years, with Fitzpatrick IV skin type. For this purpose, three areas on their lower extremities were treated using the following settings:

- IPL: 695 nm, power 15 J/cm², pulse duration 60 ms, 3 sessions at 2-week intervals
- Alexandrite laser: 755 nm, power 3 J/cm², pulse duration 2 ms, 3 sessions at 4-week intervals
- Nd:YAG laser: 1064 nm, power 32 J/cm², pulse duration 60 ms, 3 sessions at 4-week intervals

Treatment efficacy was evaluated using hair counts in the treatment area, Visual Analog Scale (VAS*), Dermatology Life Quality Index (DLQI**), and adverse event records. In terms of hair reduction, the results were distributed as follows:

- Male patient: IPL (95.1%), alexandrite laser (91.02%), and Nd:YAG laser (79.69%)
- Female patient: alexandrite laser (91.02%), Nd:YAG laser (79.69%), and IPL (20%)

A decrease in DLQI scores was observed in both patients. Hyperpigmentation and the highest VAS score (6–7) were recorded in the area treated with alexandrite laser for both patients, while Nd:YAG exhibited minimal side effects. Despite including only one participant of each sex and the limited number of sessions, this study demonstrates **the high efficacy of light-assisted hair removal as a technique for terminal hair removal. It also highlights the variation in patient sensitivity to the effects, complicating the determination of which epilation device — laser or IPL — is superior** (Sari I.W. et al., 2023).

As each option has its own advantages and limitations, the operator should understand them thoroughly and be able to adjust the exposure parameters based on the situation. Of course, the results will also depend on the hair type — the outcomes described above mainly apply to dark hair, which contains a lot of melanin. Light, red, and even gray hair is removed more effectively with the help of electric hair removal techniques.

Typically, 10 to 15 sessions at intervals of up to one month are needed to achieve good and lasting effects from light-assisted hair removal techniques, and at least 4–6 sessions are required for adequate results.

It should be emphasized that light-assisted hair removal is considered a long-term hair removal technique, not a permanent one (like

---

* The Visual Analog Scale (VAS) is a psychometric response scale that can be used in questionnaires. It is a measurement tool for subjective characteristics or attitudes that cannot be measured directly. When answering a VAS question, respondents determine their level of agreement with a statement by indicating a position along a continuous line between two endpoints.

** The Dermatology Life Quality Index (DLQI) is used by dermatologists to assess the degree of negative impact of a dermatological disease on different aspects of a patient's life, characterizing the quality of life in general: the higher the score, the lower the quality of life. The index was developed at University of Wales by Finlay A.Y. and Khan G.K. in 1993.

electrical hair removal). The damage that light causes to the hair follicle does not always lead to its death, and hair may reappear some time after a course of treatments. While it will be lighter and finer, it will continue to grow (Willey A. et al., 2007). In cases of renewed growth, it is recommended to repeat treatments every 6–12 months, or if the hair is no longer amenable to light irradiation (it has become too light and thin), removal by other techniques is indicated.

1.6.2. Effect of sex hormones on the efficacy of light-assisted hair removal in women

Laser hair removal results can be affected by various hormonal disorders and diseases such as PCOS, thyroid dysfunction, adrenal hyperplasia, hyperprolactinemia, and others. If the specialist suspects the presence of any hormonal pathology in the patient, the procedure should be postponed and the patient should be referred to a general practitioner, gynecologist, endocrinologist, or other specialized physician for evaluation. **Table II-1-5** provides a list of standardized examinations that are recommended prior to the light-assisted hair removal to reduce the risk of ineffective therapy.

We will focus on two pathologies associated with sex hormone imbalance in women — hirsutism and hyperprolactinemia.

Table II-1-5. Standard investigations before laser hair removal treatment (Arsiwala S.Z., Majid I.M., 2019)

STANDARD INVESTIGATIONS
• FSH, LH
• Thyroid function tests
• Total and free testosterone, androstenedione
• Serum DHEAS
• 17-OH progesterone
• Serum prolactin
• SHBG
• Serum cortisol
• Insulin
• Sugar
• Homo IR
• Pelvic/transvaginal USG
• Free androgen index

DHEAS: Dehydroepiandrostenedione sulfate, FSH: Follicle-stimulating hormone, LH: Luteinizing hormone, SHBG: Sex hormone-binding globulin, IR: Insulin resistance, USG: Ultrasonography.

Hirsutism

Hirsutism — excessive growth of terminal hair of the male type in women (see Part I, section 2.1) — significantly complicates the task of removing unwanted hair and can affect the effectiveness of laser hair removal (Agrawal N.K., 2013). If the patient has diseases associated with increased androgen levels (PCOS) or androgen receptor sensitivity (idiopathic hirsutism), as well as hyperprolactinemia, the primary goal is to monitor and normalize the hormonal status as part of the treatment for the underlying disease.

To achieve optimal results, laser hair removal should be performed in conjunction with hormonal therapy. Hormonal therapy for skin manifestations of hyperandrogenism enhances the effectiveness of laser hair removal and leads to the long-term cessation of hair growth. Generally, patients with hyperandrogenism require a greater number of laser hair removal treatments than those with normal hormone levels.

The effectiveness of different light-assisted hair removal techniques was evaluated in a study involving 30 hirsutism patients aged 21–50 years with III–V skin phototype (Puri N., 2015). The participants were divided into three equal groups depending on the device used:

- Group 1 (n = 10) — diode laser
- Group 2 (n = 10) — Nd:YAG laser
- Group 3 (n = 10) — IPL

The course of light-assisted hair removal consisted of 8 sessions with an interval of 4 weeks. Hair growth was evaluated in the chin area at 3-month intervals for a year. The hair removal efficacy in the three groups is shown in **Table II-1-6**.

Table II-1-6. Effectiveness of hair removal with different types of light irradiation for hirsutism (Puri N., 2015)

NUMBER OF SESSIONS	REDUCTION OF UNWANTED HAIR (%)		
	DIODE	Nd:YAG	IPL
2	40%	35%	10%
4	64%	62%	48%
8	92%	90%	70%

Undesirable phenomena were comparable in all three groups, except for pain sensations experienced during the procedure — they were minimal in the group treated with IPL and were most pronounced in the Nd:YAG group. According to the authors' conclusions, the diode laser proved to be the most effective hair elimination method for hirsutism. Although Nd:YAG was not significantly inferior in effectiveness to diode laser, its tolerability was the lowest.

Similarly, in a study by Rafi S. et al. (2024), the use of diode laser in hirsutism achieved a marked cessation of hair growth in the mandibular, chin, upper lip, and sideburn areas. According to the trichoscopy results, the average total number of hairs (terminal and vellus) per cm^2 in the foci of pathological growth after the 6th hair removal procedure decreased by 39%, and the number of terminal hairs decreased by 69%. The ratio of the number of terminal to vellus hairs decreased with repeated sessions and was statistically significant in all areas. Thus, after a course of laser epilation in patients with hirsutism there was not only a reduction in the total number of hairs in the foci of pathological growth, but also a decrease in their thickness — terminal hairs stopped growing or were replaced by vellus hairs.

The etiology of hirsutism should be considered when designing a laser hair removal regimen. In their 18-month study, Nabi N. et al. (2022) evaluated the efficacy of epilation using Nd:YAG laser in 100 female PCOS patients with hirsutism. Group A included 50 patients with idiopathic hirsutism, while Group B comprised 50 patients with hirsutism related to PCOS. The epilation course consisted of 6 sessions at 4-week intervals, followed by a 3-month observation period. After the 6th laser hair removal procedure, 70% of patients in Group A and 54% of those in Group B showed excellent results (hair reduction by more than 75%) compared to the initial level. There was a reduction in hair shaft thickness, degree of hair shaft pigmentation, the ratio of terminal to vellus hair, and hair density per cm^2. According to the analyses conducted 3 months after the 6th laser hair removal treatment, both groups experienced a decrease in these positive outcomes, which was less pronounced among the patients with idiopathic hirsutism. Thus, laser hair removal is more effective in treating idiopathic hirsutism than hirsutism caused by hyperandrogenism and PCOS.

Laser hair removal can quickly eliminate hirsutism and significantly improve patients" quality of life, but the observed improvements are temporary, as shown by Sakina S. et al. (2024). Their study included 172 female patients with PCOS and hirsutism. After a course of laser hair removal, the authors observed an initial decrease in the DLQI score along with a high level of patient satisfaction. However, most participants experienced a return of hair growth to the pre-treatment levels within 6 months, which was accompanied by a resurgence of stress disorder, anxiety, and depression symptoms. The results of this study emphasize the need to ensure that patients with hirsutism have realistic expectations regarding the long-term effects of laser hair removal.

Practical recommendations when working with women with hirsutism are as follows:

- If hirsutism manifests, the patient needs a medical examination to clarify the cause of abnormal hair growth.
- In case of hormonal disorders, laser hair removal should be carried out against the background of the primary treatment aimed at normalizing the hormone levels.
- Unwanted hair in hirsutism is less responsive to laser hair removal, so a greater number of sessions may be required to achieve a pronounced effect.
- Patients with hirsutism should realistically assess the long-term results of laser hair removal.

Hyperprolactinemia

Hyperprolactinemia is a condition characterized by increased levels of prolactin in the blood. It is commonly observed in pregnancy, persistent amenorrhea–galactorrhea syndrome, PCOS, chronic renal failure, and pituitary tumors. Hirsutism associated with hyperprolactinemia typically presents mildly, with fine and long terminal hair that has relatively low pigment levels.

Hyperprolactinemia is a significant cause of poor hair response to light exposure. Even if patients are treated, the desired effect will not be attained until the hyperprolactinemia is controlled. In these patients, prolactin levels are in the 30–90 ng/dL range, and these values indicate that, regardless of wavelength choice and device settings, acceptable results will not be possible (Agrawal N.K., 2013; Bhat Y.J. et al., 2020).

1.6.3. Light-assisted removal of red hair

Light-assisted hair removal allows practitioners to achieve permanent results, as it destroys all hair structures, including the hair follicle. However, despite the extensive study and well-described effects of radiation on biological tissues, the algorithm for selecting optimal parameters, protocols for performing the procedure, and potential complications, doctors still encounter difficulties in practice. In particular, they may struggle to adequately treat patients with red hair due to the peculiarities of their melanosomes and a genetically determined low pain threshold to thermal exposure, complicated by decreased sensitivity to anesthesia.

Color
It seems that the color intensity of red hair, and therefore the concentration of melanin in it, occupies an intermediate position between dark and light hair. It can thus be assumed that the radiation parameters for epilation in such individuals would fall between the values recommended for dark and light hair.

In the literature on light-assisted hair removal and the protocols accompanying the devices, red hair is either not discussed at all or is mentioned as an intermediate variant. However, practice shows that individuals with red hair require separate investigations and therapeutic protocols.

As a rule, red hair is even less amenable to epilation than light hair. In some cases, effective physical parameters may be impossible to identify. This may indicate that the issue lies not only in the pigment concentration but also in its composition.

We have already mentioned in Part I that melanocytes in the eumelanin follicle contain ellipsoidal (large, elongated) melanosomes with a (dense, evenly distributed) lamellar internal structure. Pheomelanogenesis is associated with melanocytes consisting of smaller spherical melanosomes, which have a less distinct internal structure where pigment granules and vesicles are diffusely arranged.

In both dark and light hair, eumelanin-type melanosomes predominate: the darker the shade, the higher their concentration. The greater the number of pheomelanosomes, the more reddish–brown the hair becomes. In fiery red hair, color develops under the influence of a rare combination of pigments — pheomelanin and erythromelanin (a special type of melanin formed by combining with iron).

Based on the presented data, one would expect that the absorption coefficient of laser radiation differs depending on the type of melanin. Although some authors have reported lower absorption coefficients of pheomelanin *in vitro* (Zonios G. et al., 2008), there are still no reliable studies that account for the differences in spectral properties of different melanin types, their percentage ratios in the target, and the thermal effect of laser radiation based on these parameters. Studies conducted in an *in vivo* animal model using Nd:YAG laser with a doubled frequency (light with a wavelength of 532 nm is well absorbed by melanin) have shown that less energy density is required for thermal degeneration of melanin in mouse skin predominantly containing epidermal eumelanin than in mouse skin predominantly containing pheomelanin (Yamaguchi H. et al., 2019). Thus, the effect of 532-nm Nd:YAG/QSw radiation on cells with different melanin subtypes was shown to differ in an *in vivo* system.

There are still no reliable methods to determine the percentage of melanin subtypes in hair, and there are no criteria for selecting physical radiation parameters for patients with red hair. In practical work, the selection of radiation parameters for red hair epilation is currently performed only empirically and does not always achieve a clinical effect.

The most likely alternative to laser removal of red hair is electrical hair removal. This technique also aims to destroy the hair follicle and suppresses hair growth for a long period. However, it is a highly painful procedure that compromises skin integrity, so red-haired patients rarely agree to electrical hair removal.

Pain

Another factor contributing to the difficulty of laser hair removal is the increased skin sensitivity of red-haired people. Pain sensitivity is linked to the *MC1R* type.

Individuals with pale skin and red hair possess a mutation in the *MC1R* gene that is also linked to altered heat receptor pain sensitivity. Studies have demonstrated that this group tends to be exceptionally sensitive to both cold and heat, and red-haired women require a higher dosage of anesthesia than their dark-haired counterparts to achieve an analgesic effect (Andresen T. et al., 2011). Due to their lower pain threshold, these patients are more likely to decline follow-up sessions because of intense pain sensations. Additionally, the use of analgesics is often ineffective due to their genetically determined reduced sensitivity to local anesthetics.

Still, this does not mean that red-haired patients are unsuitable for laser hair removal and should immediately refuse the procedure. Instead, the doctor should explain all possible difficulties to ensure that the patient has realistic expectations. Second, it is essential to be as attentive as possible in choosing the laser exposure parameters.

To make a more accurate individual prognosis for each red-haired patient, a test hair removal procedure should be conducted on a small sample in the area of the proposed treatment during the initial consultation, using the radiation parameters expected to provide a clinical effect. Changes such as hair whitening and curling during the test procedure indicate the clinical effectiveness of laser exposure and allow the practitioner to start laser therapy. If there is no result, the patient should not proceed with the treatment due to its ineffectiveness for their hair color.

1.7. Safety issues

1.7.1. Contraindications to light-assisted hair removal

Absolute contraindications:
- Acute and chronic skin diseases
- Decompensated stages of diabetes mellitus
- Varicose veins at the site of the procedure
- Severe forms of hypertension and ischemic heart disease
- Acute forms of herpes
- Infectious diseases
- Keloid disease
- Skin malignancies

Relative contraindications:
- Pregnancy
- Mental illness

The range of **specific** contraindications to light-assisted hair removal techniques is limited to hypersensitivity to sunlight (photodermatosis).

1.7.2. Photosensitizers that increase the risk of burn injury

The likelihood of burns and post-inflammatory hyperpigmentation increases if patients are taking drugs with photosensitizing properties (**Table II-1-7**).

Table II-1-7. Some drugs that cause photosensitization

GROUP OF MEDICINES	DRUGS
Antimicrobials	• Amoxicillin • Griseofulvin • Doxycycline • Minocycline • Oxytetracycline • Sulfonamides • Tetracycline • Trimethoprim
Non-steroidal anti-inflammatory drugs (NSAIDs)	• Diclofenac • Ibuprofen • Indomethacin • Piroxicam • Fenbufen • Phenylbutazone
Antidepressants	• Amitriptyline • Fluoxetine
Antihistamines (H_1- and H_2-histamine receptor blockers)	• Ranitidine • Cimetidine
Hypotensive agents	• Methyldopa • Nifedipine

Parsnip, parsley, celery juice, and freshly squeezed citrus juices can increase skin sensitivity to light, both when applied to the skin and when consumed orally. Figs, rose petal jam, and spicy foods sometimes have the same effect.

Various herbs used in phytotherapy and dietary supplements — St. John's wort, clover, milkweed, tansy, turpentine, and anchovy — can lead to undesirable skin reactions to radiation. The problem is that, as the composition of dietary supplements may not coincide with the declared composition, it is not always possible to predict in advance how the skin will react to UV exposure.

1.7.3. Nevi in the area of light-assisted hair removal

The nevus is composed of melanocytes and is characterized by a high melanin content. For this reason, photons of light radiation used for epilation can be absorbed by nevus melanocytes with subsequent thermal tissue damage (Garrido-Rios A.A. et al., 2013). Several such cases have been described in the literature. According to the review of scientific publications performed by Dessinioti C. et al. (2023), clinical changes in 20.2–100% of nevi in 20–59% of patients are noted after light-assisted hair removal.

Clinical and morphological changes in the nevi in the treatment area are most often inflammatory, including edema, redness, wetting, ulceration, and crust formation. Heterogeneity and changes in pigmentation intensity, as well as nevus regression, are also possible (Acle R. et al., 2022). The observed changes are typically characteristic manifestations of thermal damage. However, given the presence of melanocytes in the area of exposure, there is a risk of malignant degeneration of the pigmentary formation over time. Clinical changes in pigmentary formations following light-assisted hair removal correspond to the criterion "E" (evolution) of the international system of diagnostic criteria ABCDE (asymmetry, uneven borders, color and size changes, heterogeneity, diameter >6 mm). This system of criteria has long been used for the visual detection of melanoma (Tsao H. et al., 2015).

There are objective diagnostic techniques to assess nevus changes. These include:

- Dermoscopy, including sequential digital dermoscopy with visualization to identify suspicious neoplasms by observing them over time
- Reflectance confocal microscopy
- Histological examination

Dermoscopic evaluation of nevus changes after light-assisted hair removal

Three prospective studies involving 79 participants and several case reports focus on atypical dermoscopic changes in pigmented neoplasms after laser treatment (Boleira M. et al., 2015; Guicciardi F. et al., 2019; Acle R. et al., 2022; Nasimi M. et al., 2022). The described atypical changes were only characteristic of nevi located on treated body sites and were not observed in nevi on intact control sites. In published prospective studies, the following dermoscopic changes in pigmented neoplasms were most commonly noted (**Fig. II-1-8**):

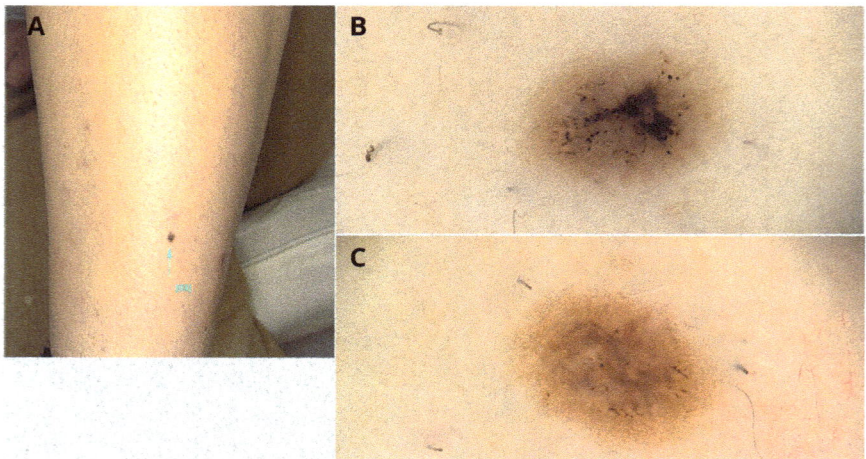

Figure II-1-8. Female, 36 years old. Dermoscopic changes of pigmented lesions after light-assisted hair removal (adapted from Dessinioti C. et al., 2023)

An atypical pigmented lesion was noted on the front of the left lower leg in a 36-year-old woman who had undergone laser hair removal on her legs 3 weeks prior. (A) Clinical aspect. (B) Dermoscopy shows loss of the pigment network, a central dark brownish blotch, and a gray structureless area. (C) At the 2-week follow-up (5 weeks after the laser hair removal), a reticular pigment network is starting to become evident at the periphery. A gray area is still seen in the center of the lesion.

- Discoloration
- Crusting
- Changes in the pattern of the pigment network, including gray and blue areas, gray dots/globules, and whitish structureless areas

Dermoscopic changes in nevi after light-assisted hair removal depend on the time of evaluation and may become more prominent (**Fig. II-1-9**).

One alarming symptom is the appearance of a new nevus after light-assisted hair removal that does not resemble the pigmented masses already present (Boleira M. et al., 2015).

Differential diagnosis

A two-stage diagnostic algorithm facilitates therapeutic protocol selection according to the type of mass (Marghoob A.A., Braun R., 2010).

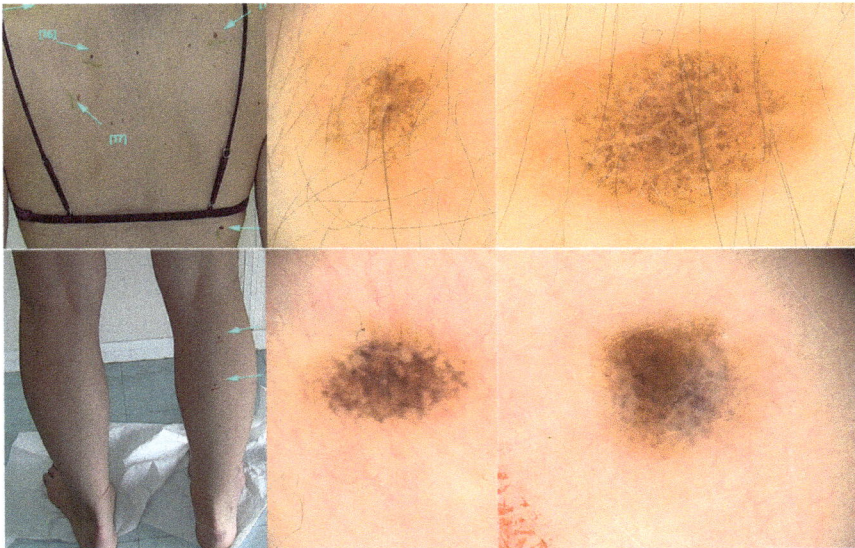

Figure II-1-9. The same woman at her follow-up visit (adapted from Dessinioti C. et al., 2023)

Upper panel: Nevi on her back that had not undergone laser hair removal showing a globular pigment network. Lower panel: Lesions on the right calf that had undergone laser hair removal showing persistent changes 5 weeks after photoepilation. Dermoscopy reveals loss of the pigment network and loss of pigmentation, which is particularly evident in one half of the nevus. Grayish areas are also observed in one half of the nevus.

- The first step is to differentially diagnose non-melanocytic neoplasms (seborrheic keratosis, vascular neoplasm, basal cell carcinoma) and melanocytic neoplasms.
- In the second step, melanocytic masses are categorized into benign and malignant (melanoma).

In cases where it is difficult to determine the type of mass (melanocytic or non-melanocytic), to avoid missing skin cancer, the mass is classified as "structureless" and considered suspected melanoma. The presence of white and blue areas, along with pigmentation resembling a blue–white veil, indicates an increased risk of malignant degeneration of the pigmented mass.

The presence of clinical and dermoscopic changes, including signs of atypia, in a pigmented neoplasm after light-assisted hair removal requires immediate differential diagnosis between benign pigmented neoplasm and melanoma. For this purpose, sequential digital dermoscopy, reflectance confocal microscopy (if available), and histological examination of biopsy specimens or the neoplasm itself after surgical excision are used.

Presumably, histological changes consistent with thermal destruction of melanocytes, nevus cells, surrounding keratinocytes, and stromal matrix include subepidermal blister formation, deformed or fragmented melanocytes in the epidermis or at the dermal–epidermal junction, and homogenization of collagen in the papillary dermis (Soden C.E. et al., 2001).

Dermoscopic features such as the presence of brown pigment flecks without a melanocytic pattern correlate with the presence of superficial microcrustules in histological examination. Lesions accompanied by central whitish areas detected during dermoscopy have been histologically characterized by fibrosis in the papillary layer of the dermis and regression phenomena. Histopathologically, blue color corresponds to the melanin of melanophages or pigmented melanocytes in the dermis. Melanophages are often found in gray areas during histological examination.

How to protect pigmented lesions during light-assisted hair removal treatment

The presence of changes in nevi located on areas of the body that have undergone light-assisted hair removal compared to nevi on untreated areas confirms the possibility of the effect of light radiation on the structural and functional state of nevi. **Nonetheless, it should be noted that no clinical cases of melanoma development after laser or IPL epilation have been described in known scientific publications.**

According to the European Society of Laser Dermatology (ESLD) guidelines, pigmented nevi should be avoided or covered with white adhesive tape during light-assisted hair removal procedures (Drosner M., Adatto M., 2005). A white kajal pencil containing titanium dioxide is widely used in many countries but may not be sufficient to protect nevi. Bodendorf M.O. et al. (2013) tested the ability of different materials to absorb radiation from diode (808 nm, 30 J/cm^2, 12 ms) and alexandrite (755 nm, 30 J/cm^2, 40 ms) lasers. The tested materials were applied to clear glass, and the researchers evaluated the light transmission decrement compared to clear glass. For diode and alexandrite lasers, respectively, transmittance decreased:

- to 8.77% and 7.99% when zinc oxide paste (1 g/cm^2) was applied
- to 8.05% and 3.62% when using a wooden spatula as a screen
- to 19.85% and 16.91% when sunscreen was applied
- to 19.25% and 20.78% when applying polyurethane foam
- to 76.43% and 71.03% after the application of white kajal pencil

Zinc paste and a wooden spatula demonstrated the best absorption properties; however, wood-based screens are not recommended for nevus protection due to the risk of fire associated with repeated laser applications (Bodendorf M.O. et al., 2013).

The application of zinc paste to the melanocytic nevi in sufficient quantities protected the nevi from thermal damage during laser hair removal (**Fig. II-1-10**). This cost-effective and efficient technique avoids undesirable events during light-assisted hair removal in the area where the nevi are located.

In conclusion, clinical and dermoscopic changes and signs of atypia have been observed in melanocytic masses after light-assisted hair

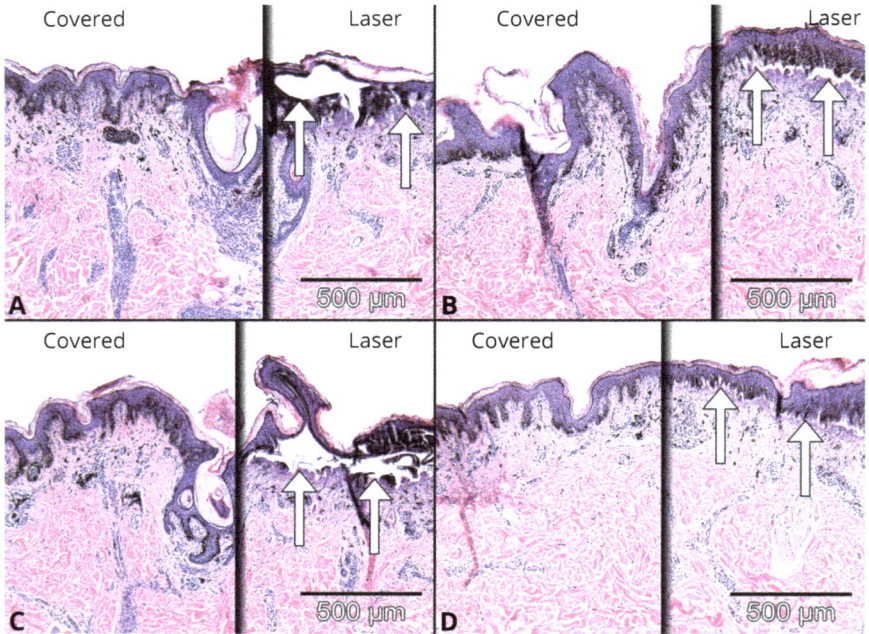

Figure II-1-10. Histological changes after a single pass with alexandrite laser (30 J/cm^2, 40 ms) on a congenital nevus half-covered with (A) zinc paste, (B) polyurethane foam, (C) sunscreen, and (D) wooden spatula (adapted from Bodendorf M.O. et al., 2013)

removal, necessitating follow-up evaluation by digital dermoscopy or histological examination to establish an unequivocal diagnosis. As these diagnostic approaches can be time-consuming and distressing for the patient, it is critical to prevent exposure of pigmented lesions to radiation during the procedure.

1.8. Peculiarities of light-assisted hair removal procedures

Before the session

Before performing light-assisted hair removal, it is necessary to collect a medical history. If there are contraindications (see Part II, section 1.7.1), the procedure should not be performed. In addition, the following information should be noted:

- Endocrine disorders or menstrual disorders should attract the attention of a specialist as such conditions may be the cause of hirsutism
- If lanugo-type hypertrichosis develops suddenly, paraneoplastic syndrome should be suspected
- Recurrent herpetic infection around the mouth or in the genital area requires prophylactic treatment with valacyclovir 10–14 days before a light-assisted therapy session

During the preliminary consultation, it is essential to inform the patient about possible undesirable reactions, set realistic expectations, and discuss the treatment costs. The patient should understand that multiple sessions may be necessary, but even this does not guarantee stable hair removal, as some regrowth can occur after a few years. A single treatment typically results in slower hair growth for 2–6 months.

Patients should also know that the hair will not fall out immediately but will become thinner over a few days or weeks. It should be explained that sun exposure should be avoided after the procedure, as hyper- or hypopigmentation foci may develop.

All other hair removal techniques should be avoided 2–4 weeks prior to light-assisted hair removal, as they eliminate the target for light exposure. However, a few days or immediately before the treatment, the hair should be shaved to prevent thermolysis of the regrown hair shafts from causing skin burns.

During the session

Local anesthesia can be used before light-assisted hair removal. The amount and type of drug is selected depending on the treated area and the patient's pain threshold. When working in sensitive areas, such as the upper lip and bikini area, a longer exposure to anesthetic may be needed — typically 30–60 minutes. Other pain suppression options include ice, air blowing, local infiltration anesthesia, and regional nerve block.

It is crucial to adequately protect the eyes — both the patient's and the operator's (and, if there are outside observers, their eyes as well). Protective goggles are chosen based on the type of radiation; thus, IPL goggles cannot be used when working with lasers, and vice versa.

At the beginning of the procedure, a test flash is performed on a small, inconspicuous area of skin. The presence of perifollicular edema or slight skin redness can serve as a criterion for correctly setting the equipment. It is advisable to avoid working in areas with pigment spots and tattoos to prevent burns.

After the session

Although most modern lasers and IPL devices have built-in cooling systems, ice packs or cooling agents can be used after the procedure to minimize pain and swelling. Redness and slight swelling after the procedure are normal, and the patient should be warned about this in advance. If burns occur, topical steroids of sufficient strength should be applied immediately and continued for several days. Antibiotics can be prescribed if necessary.

It is mandatory to use sunscreen during the sunny season. For more information on skincare after hair removal, see Part II, Ch. 6.

1.9. Effect on axillary skin microbiome and sweat odor

Due to the secretions of eccrine, apocrine, and sebaceous glands, the axillae provide a moist and nutrient-rich habitat for a large population of microorganisms. The appearance of odorous sweat is caused by the biotransformation of naturally occurring odorless secretions into volatile odorous molecules. Can light-assisted hair removal in the underarm area not only remove hair, but also reduce the odor of sweat? As it turns out, yes.

The microbiome of the axillary skin is dominated by *Staphylococcus aureus*, *Corynebacterium*, and *Propionibacterium*. These microorganisms create ecological competition against pathogenic bacteria and help prevent their spread. The hydrolysis of sebum lipids by the commensal flora produces free fatty acids that are toxic to many pathogens. Thus, a healthy microbiome protects the skin from infectious inflammatory diseases (Taylor D. et al., 2003). During the biotransformation of sebum components, volatile substances responsible for the odor of sweat are also formed; coryneform bacteria are the main contributors to their appearance (James A.G. et al., 2013).

The impact of laser hair removal on the composition of the axillary microbiome and the severity of sweat odor was examined in several studies.

Fazel Z. et al. (2020) evaluated microbiome changes after laser hair removal in 30 healthy women. The average age of the participants was 30 years. Participants were asked to avoid using deodorants, as well as antifungal or antibacterial cleansers in the axillae throughout the study. An alexandrite laser (755 nm) was used for hair removal. All patients underwent 6 laser hair removal treatments at 4- to 6-week intervals. For the first 3 procedures, the following laser treatment parameters were used: 18 mm spot size, 3 ms pulse duration, and 10 J/cm^2 radiation density. During the last 3 treatments, the energy density was increased to 14 J/cm^2. After the 3rd and 6th treatments, a microbiological study of the microbiome composition was performed. Sweat odor severity was evaluated using the "improvement," "worsening," and "no change" criteria.

The average number of bacterial colonies before laser hair removal was 17.97×10^6. After the 3rd hair removal treatment, the rate decreased to 17.72×10^6, and after the 6th treatment, it declined to 17.26×10^6. These results demonstrate that the total number of bacteria after laser treatment does not decrease significantly. However, the effect of laser treatment on the microbiome representatives was quite different: after laser treatment, there was a decrease in the number of *Micrococcus luteus* (*M. luteus*) and *Staphylococcus aureus* (*S. aureus*) and an increase in the number of *Staphylococcus epidermidis* (*S. epidermidis*).

The majority of participants reported a decrease in sweat odor by the end of the laser hair removal course. A reduction in sweat odor intensity ("improvement") was observed in 19 patients (63.3%), no change in 6 patients (20%), and a worsening in 5 patients (16.7%).

In patients where sweat odor intensity declined, the *S. epidermidis* strain prevailed, whereas *M. luteus* and *S. aureus* were the most abundant in cases of aggravation and no change, respectively. Different results were obtained by Elsaeed Eldeeb M. et al. (2024) as part of their study focusing on changes in the skin microbiome and the severity of sweat odor after laser hair removal in the axillary region. Their study sample comprised 30 women with a mean age of 26 years. Nd:YAG laser (spot size 15–18 mm, energy flux density 24–35 J/cm^2, pulse duration 30–40 ms) was used for axillary epilation. *Staphylococcus hominis* (*S. hominis*) was the predominant species in all participants before and after laser hair removal. There was a significant decrease in mean colony counts (CFU/cm^2) for total aerobes (27.89 vs. 12.63×10^6), total anaerobes (33.87 vs. 10.37×10^6), and total staphylococci (24.85 vs. 10.50×10^6). Additionally, there was a non-significant decrease in the mean number of lipophilic bacteria and *S. hominis*. No significant decrease in the *S. epidermidis*, *S. saprophyticus*, and *S. aureus* quantities was observed, likely due to the smaller number of colonies of these species isolated during this study.

Regarding sweat odor, by the end of the study, 12 participants (40%) reported an increase, 2 (6.7%) noted a decrease, and 16 (53.3%) experienced no change. The predominant bacterial strain among those with increased and decreased sweat odor was *S. hominis*. Additionally, a significant correlation was observed between the increase in sweat odor and the decrease in total aerobes, anaerobes, staphylococci, and *S. hominis*.

The reviewed studies indicate a pronounced effect of laser treatment on the axillary microbiome. The nature of this effect may depend on the energy density and the structural properties of the microorganism's membrane. It is unclear whether laser treatment independently enhances the growth of a specific strain of bacteria or whether its inhibitory effect on certain strains creates better conditions for the growth of a particular strain. Conversely, differences in the response to laser irradiation among various bacterial species stem from genomic mutations or changes in their membrane.

Be that as it may, the **use of laser radiation in the axillary region for the purpose of removing unwanted hair induces changes in the microbial flora, thus reducing the severity of sweat odor**.

1.10. Side effects of light-assisted hair removal

Skin phototype, the anatomical area that is exposed, and contact with sunlight before the procedure all affect the likelihood of side effects after the procedure. Sun-protected areas (underarms and bikini area) are less prone to problems than exposed skin.

Most commonly occurring issues in the treatment area are:

- Erythema
- Swelling
- Blisters
- Transient telangiectasia
- Scaling
- Itching
- Pain
- Hyperpigmentation

Generally, adverse reactions resolve quickly; however, in the case of a burn, persistent dyschromia and scarring may form.

Rarely occurring adverse effects include (Rasheed A.I., 2009; Mallat F. et al., 2023):

- Acne exacerbation
- Rosacea-like rash
- Herpetic infection exacerbation
- Premature hair graying
- Hair ingrowth into the skin
- Paradoxical hypertrichosis
- Hyperhidrosis
- Long-lasting diffuse redness and edema of the facial skin
- Inflammatory and pigmentary changes to existing nevi and age spots
- Fox–Fordyce disease (a chronic disease of the apocrine glands, manifested by itchy skin rashes in the axillae, pubic area, and around the nipples)

Depending on the power of radiation, light can cause various photobiological effects — both thermal (destructive) and biological (stimulating). If the radiation power is insufficient, the risk of unpredictable effects (including increased hair growth) due to the initiation of a whole range of biological processes rises. Conversely, excessive radiation power can result in skin burns. The possibility of burns also increases when taking photosensitizing drugs (see Part II, section 1.7.2).

In some cases, laser hair removal causes the opposite reaction — a paradoxical increase in hair growth (**paradoxical hypertrichosis**). Even if hair follicles are mostly destroyed, it is likely that parts of them can persist, regenerate and, in the presence of excess androgens, facilitate strong growth of terminal pigmented hair. This may explain why some women experience paradoxical hypertrichosis after light-assisted hair removal. This condition occurs more often on darker skin and/or after exposure to laser light of low energy density. The most common sites for paradoxical hypertrichosis are the chin and neck, with excessive hair growth reported in 6–10% of cases (Alajlan A. et al., 2005). Paradoxical hypertrichosis is treated with further laser hair removal sessions at high energy densities and with short pulses. It is important to ensure adequate cooling of the patient's skin to prevent burns.

Very rarely, persistent urticaria occurs in patients who have previously tolerated the procedure easily and have no history of urticaria. This phenomenon is still poorly understood, and its pathogenesis remains unclear. It is likely an allergic reaction to cryogen or sensitivity to certain radiation wavelengths. Prolonged hyperhidrosis can also occur after the procedure in the armpit area, most often when using Nd:YAG laser, which does not destroy but stimulates the sweat glands (Aydin F. et al., 2009).

Eye damage should not be overlooked, given that when using wavelengths in the visible range (400–720 nm) or close to IR part of the spectrum (720–1400 nm), eye exposure to the laser beam can cause retinal burns and reduced vision. Therefore, without exception, both the patient and the specialist should wear protective eyewear. Laser hair removal should not be performed on eyebrows and eyelids, as there are reports of severe eye damage in this case (cataracts, iritis, iris atrophy, etc.).

Choosing the right lasers and IPL systems with individualized parameters for each patient is crucial, especially for individuals with darker skin tones. Most complications can be avoided by selecting a laser suitable for the patient's phototype, correctly adjusting the energy flux density and spot size, and employing appropriate cooling methods. Therefore, it is essential that light-assisted hair removal procedures are carried out by trained personnel who possess a solid understanding of laser mechanisms, the technology involved, and the complications that may arise during treatment.

1.11. At-home light-assisted hair removal

Light-assisted hair removal devices for at-home use are becoming increasingly common (Kaliyadan F. et al., 2022). These devices work on the same principle as professional high-energy lasers and IPL systems, but their energy levels are much lower, so the efficiency of photothermal destruction of follicles is also low. Nevertheless, the delivered radiation is still selectively absorbed by melanin of the hair shaft and HF, causing various processes affecting hair growth in these structures.

In a study by Town G. et al. (2019), a single low-energy-density pulse from both an 810 nm diode laser (6.6 J/cm^2, 16 ms) and an IPL device (9 J/cm^2, 15 ms and 6.8 J/cm^2, 1.9 ms) for home use was shown to result in the induction of a hair transition from the anagen to catagen state. The catagen transition was characterized by morphological changes similar to those occurring *in vivo*, with isolated apoptosis events in dermal papillae and HF outer root sheath cells (van Vlimmeren M.A.A. et al., 2019). Thus, "smooth skin" can be expected after home treatments due to synchronized loss of treated hair, and regular sessions could theoretically lead to HF miniaturization due to cumulative effects on dermal papilla and outer root sheath cells. Notably, different studies suggest that hair reduction results comparable to those yielded by professional devices can be attained, but only if the equipment is used regularly. When treatments are discontinued, hair growth resumes fairly quickly.

In a cross-sectional study by Kaliyadan F. et al. (2022), 39 of 111 participating individuals used light-assisted hair removal devices at home, and only 4 reported adverse reactions, including redness, puffiness, burns, and discoloration in the treatment area.

An interesting point to note here is the lack of data on the paradoxical increase in hair growth after at-home light treatments, as opposed
to the professional ones. Scientists suggest that this unpleasant effect of high-energy hair removal may be primarily due to inflammation in response to damage, rather than heating (to low temperatures)
(Town G., Bjerring P., 2016).

Some hair removal devices currently on the market have received
FDA approval for at-home use, such as Silk'n and Veet (Home Inno-
vations), Tria (Tria Beauty), Remington and LumaRx (Shaser), Lumea
(Philips), etc.

Chapter 2
Electrical hair removal

Electrical hair removal involves irreversible destruction of the hair follicle with the help of electric current. It is the oldest epilation method. As early as 1875 Charles Michel used electrolysis to remove ingrown eyelashes (trichiasis). In 1924, Henri Baudier proposed the thermolysis technique, and in 1945, Arthur Hinkel and Henry St. Pierre "combined" them into the blend.

Electrical hair removal is approved by the FDA as a "permanent hair removal technique." Its principle is based on the capacity of electric current to heat the tissue through which it passes. Its main advantage is its versatility, as it can be used to remove almost any hair. However, the effectiveness of electrical hair removal is highly dependent on the professionalism and experience of the specialist performing the procedure. Additionally, the treatment speed is slow, as a relatively large number of sessions is needed to achieve a lasting effect (typically, 10 to 15 sessions with 30-day intervals between them). Thus, patients should be aware that a successful final result will require a great deal of patience, time, and money.

There are two technological options for performing electrical hair removal:

1. **With a needle** (electrolysis, thermolysis, and their modifications — blend, sequential blend, flush, sequential flush) **(Fig. II-2-1)**
2. **Using forceps (Fig. II-2-2)**

Currently, needle epilation techniques are recognized as the primary options for electrical hair removal. The needle is the active electrode to which the electric current is applied, while the passive electrode, essential for closing the electric circuit, is fixed on the patient's body. This means that the human body itself is a crucial component of the electrical circuit that conducts the current. Although this process is safe,

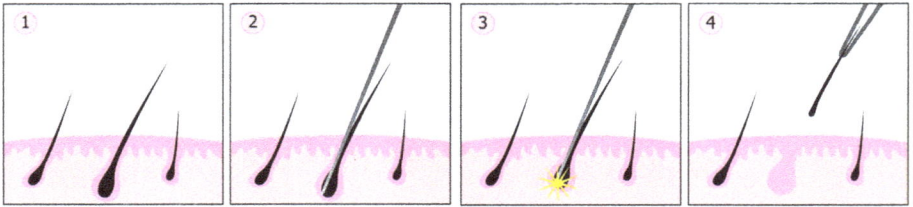

Figure II-2-1. General diagram of electric needle hair removal

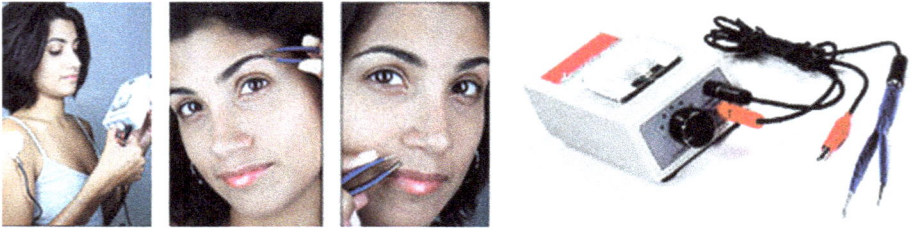

Figure II-2-2. Electric hair removal with tweezers

as demonstrated by various physiotherapy electro procedures, certain limitations exist, namely the presence of:

- Implants, pacemakers, reinforced threads, and intrauterine devices
- Cardiovascular failure
- Neoplasms
- Fevers
- Open wounds
- Systemic skin disease
- Pregnancy

In terms of indications, electrical hair removal can be used to remove hair of any color and any localization (except nasal hair). In addition, electrical hair removal can be combined with the administration of pharmacological preparations by electrophoresis (for example, to restore pH, to relieve swelling and irritation that may appear after the procedure). Alternatively, special solutions or gels that inhibit hair growth can be injected into the hair canals (this technique is called **epilsoft**). Several epilsoft sessions can achieve hair thinning, while also reducing the number of hairs. Taking into account the stages of hair growth, procedures can be carried out every 20–30 days for a long time. The best results are achieved when thin hair is treated.

2.1. Electrolysis

Electrolysis (galvanic epilation) is the most popular technique of hair removal using electric current. This is confirmed by the fact that in some popular reference books the terms "electrical hair removal" and "electrolysis" are treated as synonyms.

The technique relies on the electrochemical action of galvanic current, which is a **constant unidirectional current** of low strength and intensity. During the procedure, the current is delivered through a thin needle that is inserted into the skin to the depth of the hair follicle, where the hair growth zone is destroyed. The needle inserted into the hair follicle connects to the negative pole while the positive (passive) electrode is attached to the forearm or shin, or simply placed in the patient's hand.

Under the action of the current in the hair follicle tissue, there is a movement of charged ions to the poles of opposite sign. Namely, positively charged ions of tissue medium (Na^+ and K^+) move to the negative electrode, the excessive amount of which is compensated by negatively charged ions (OH^-), which leads to strong alkalinization of the medium due to local accumulation of NaOH and KOH. A strongly alkaline environment causes the death of hair follicle cells, depriving the HF of the ability to regenerate.

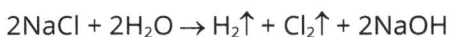

$$2NaCl + 2H_2O \rightarrow H_2\uparrow + Cl_2\uparrow + 2NaOH$$

It is important to note that these reactions take place in a saline solution. The more of it there is, the more alkaline it is, and therefore, the more pronounced the epilating effect will be. Consequently, **galvanic epilation should preferably be performed on pre-moisturized skin**.

The amount of alkali produced is also influenced by the current strength: the higher the current, the more alkali is generated, and the greater the pain experienced during the procedure. An alternative option is to use a lower current for a more extended period. The choice of a particular mode depends on the patient's sensitivity to pain. Usually, the procedure is started at low levels and the current is gradually increased until it is possible to easily extract the hair from the follicle.

The advantage of this technique is that if areas of the hair follicle are out of reach of the needle, the resulting alkali is distributed throughout the follicle. The disadvantage is that it takes quite a long time to remove the hair, averaging around 10 seconds per hair, while treating thick or curly hair can take up to a minute.

Electrolysis is a less painful and less risky hair removal technique than thermolysis (see Part II, section 2.2). However, even though multi-needle systems have been used recently, the procedure takes a long time to complete.

Principle	Destruction of the hair follicle by a chemical reaction that occurs at the end of the needle electrode when a direct electric current is passed. The resulting alkali and acid destroy the cells. The procedure is carried out as follows: one electrode is held in the patient's hand, the other electrode (needle) is brought to the hair follicle. The sign of follicle destruction is foam, which appears at the mouth of the hair. The hair is then removed with tweezers.
Advantages	• Not as painful as thermolysis (see Part II, section 2.2) • Most patients tolerate the procedure well • High hair removal rate in one treatment • Gives the opportunity to destroy the follicle and bulge area, even if there is no precise needle hit — due to the impregnation of tissues with alkali
Disadvantages	Longer procedure than thermolysis (treatment speed is 2–6 hairs per minute)
Complications	Minor burns and subsequent scarring cannot be ruled out
Results	Usually, visible effect is achieved from the first session. However, since a small area can be treated in one session, it is necessary to carry out several sessions.

2.2. Thermolysis

As its name suggests, thermolysis is a technique of tissue destruction by heat. It is based on the action of **alternating current of high frequency** (1.3, 5, 13.56, and 27.12 MHz) and low voltage. The current is also delivered through a thin needle that is inserted into the skin to the depth of the HF, where localized heating occurs with coagulation of the hair papilla and destruction of the follicle (Kim D.H. et al., 2015). Heating is realized due to a constant change of orientation of water molecules, which are dipoles (their rotation), and charged particles, with a frequency corresponding to the current frequency. Accordingly, the higher the current frequency, the faster the heating process.

Thermolysis is a painful procedure, so many patients need local anesthesia (lidocaine, novocaine, trimecaine, etc.). However, the liquid anesthetics can significantly affect the parameters of the procedure, reducing its effectiveness. There is also a risk of further formation of small atrophic scars, folliculitis, and even local septic manifestations.

Principle	Destruction of follicle cells under the action of local heating caused by alternating electric current, which is brought to the hair follicle with a thin needle. The skin is pre-treated with an anesthetic preparation.
Advantages	• Obtaining a lasting effect • Faster than electrolysis (10–35 hairs per minute)
Disadvantages	• Small target area — it is very easy to insert the needle tip past the hair follicle. This is particularly a problem for curly hair or hair that has been previously removed by plucking. In these cases, the HF and the hair papilla may not be directly aligned. • Pain, which cannot always be eliminated with local anesthesia. Anesthetic injections are not desirable, as this reduces the procedure effectiveness. • Due to painfulness, it is difficult to perform the procedure in highly sensitive areas (face, underarms, bikini area).
Complications	• There may be scarring • Irritation may occur
Results	The hair follicle is not always destroyed the first time. Multiple sessions are required.

Thermolysis
destruction by
current through
heating

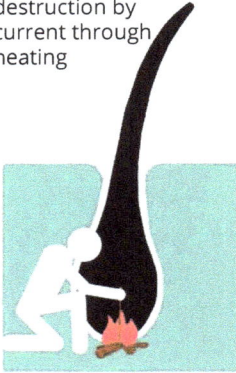

Electrolysis
destruction by
current through
chemical
reaction

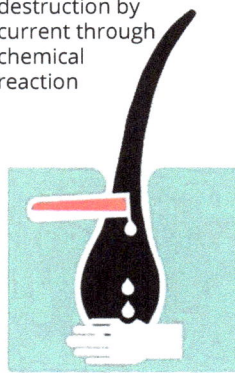

Figure II-2-3.
Comparison of
electric hair removal
by thermolysis and
electrolysis

Each of these techniques has its advantages and disadvantages (**Fig. II-2-3**). As noted previously, improved modifications of electrical hair removal have been developed to enhance the former and reduce the latter.

2.3. Blend

Blend epilation combines the effects of alternating (thermolysis) and direct (electrolysis) electric currents on the hair follicle. This technique relies on the principle that the heat generated during thermolysis speeds up the electrolysis process. Consequently, it is possible to reduce the exposure time necessary for producing the required amount of sodium hydroxide (NaOH) by 2–4 times, averaging at ≈ 5 s. As a result, this technique provides the advantages of both traditional thermolysis (rapid exposure) and electrolysis (less painful experience). Due to the dual impact on the HF, the likelihood of its complete destruction is greater than that of classical electrical hair removal techniques. However, the blend technique inherits not only the advantages but also the disadvantages of its predecessors — the procedure speed remains relatively slow, and the risk of scarring and folliculitis is higher than desired.

2.4. Sequential blend

Sequential blend is an improved blend technique. The improvement is that, to enhance the effect of HF destruction during needle insertion, the amplitude of direct current is reduced at the moment of impulse. This reduction decreases painful sensations while providing a more intense effect on the follicle.

2.5. Flash

The flash technique is an improved version of thermolysis that uses high-frequency alternating current (2 MHz) and the duration of exposure per hair is extremely short (0.01–0.09 s). As a result, heat dissipation to the surrounding tissue is significantly lower, so this technique is less painful and faster than the classic version (**Fig. II-2-4**). However, it can only be performed by a skilled specialist. In addition, programs offered by different manufacturers exhibit some notable variations — for example, microflash (0.001 s) and multiplex (combination of conventional thermolysis [0.5–2.5 s] and microflash pulse). In general, the double pulse mode is used quite often, as one pulse is aimed at destroying the hair papilla, and the other targets the bulge.

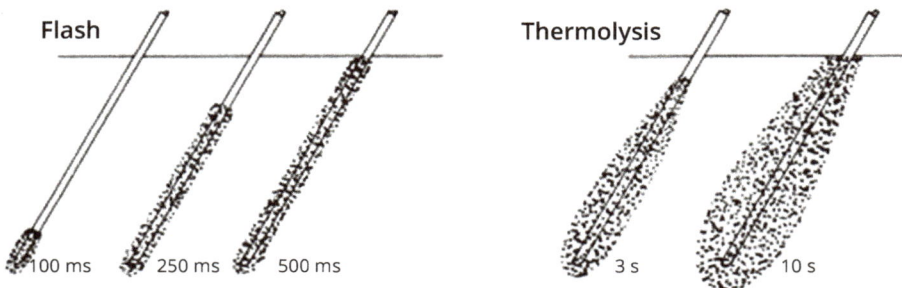

Figure II-2-4. Comparison of the thermal effects of the flash technique and classical thermolysis (adapted from Hinkel A.R., Lind R.W., 1968)

2.6. Sequential flash

Sequential flash is an advanced technique of flash thermolysis that uses a high-frequency sinusoidal current and varies the time of exposure to the hair. This speeds up the hair removal process and allows the mode of operation to be tailored to specific hair texture.

2.7. Tweezerman-assisted electrical hair removal

The tweezing technique appeared later than the needle epilation variants, in 1959. According to the manufacturers' claims, its principle of operation is based on capturing a hair shaft with special tweezers and passing an electric current through them for several minutes to transfer electrical energy to heat the HF. However, hair is a dielectric by its structure and practically does not conduct electric current. The skin surrounding it, on the other hand, is a current conductor, albeit a weak one. As a result, the current transmitted to the hair shaft is more likely to disperse through the skin. Still, despite many questions about its effectiveness, this technique is safe and painless.

On the other hand, the procedures are very time-consuming, as a few minutes may be spent on a single hair. In 1985, the American Trade Commission banned the sale of electric tweezers relying on alternating current. The ban was based on numerous consumer complaints about the lack of the claimed "permanent hair removal." Although the company that manufactured the devices subsequently commissioned studies to confirm their efficacy, in 1998, after reviewing them, the FDA concluded that the reported results did not support their claimed ability to provide "permanent hair removal." However, tweezing devices, including those based on the use of direct current (galvanic tweezers), can still be found on the market.

Chapter 3
Ultrasonic hair removal

The term "ultrasonic hair removal" is usually understood as a complex intervention, the first stage of which is waxing. The technique owes its name to the second part, when after waxing, the skin surface is treated with special compositions, the molecules and ions of which are delivered to the deep dermal layers with the help of ultrasonic action. Here, they inhibit (slow down) the germ cell division process and even partially destroy the hair follicle due to the alkaline pH value.

The ultrasonic hair removal technique can be very effective when a particular hair unit is highly sensitive to the inhibitors used.

3.1. Mechanism of action

Any device designed to increase skin permeability (sonophoresis) can be used for ultrasonic hair removal.

Sonophoresis (syn.: phonophoresis; from Latin *sonus* — sound, Greek *phōnē* — sound, voice, Greek *phoresis* — carrying, transfer) is a transdermal drug delivery technique based on the use of ultrasound to increase the permeability of the *stratum corneum*.

According to the frequencies used, we distinguish:
1. **Low-frequency sonophoresis (LFS)** at 20–100 kHz
2. **High-frequency sonophoresis (HFS)** at 0.7–16 MHz (a range that includes both therapeutic and high-frequency ultrasound waves, but frequencies between 1 and 3 MHz are generally used)

The mechanisms by which medium-frequency ultrasonic waves (ranging from approximately 100 to 700 kHz) facilitate the transdermal transport of active substances have not been sufficiently studied;

therefore, waves of this frequency are not included in any of the afore-mentioned groups.

Both HFS and LFS enhance the penetration of various substances through the skin, but their mechanisms of action are different. The mechanisms of increasing skin permeability under the action of ultrasound are divided into two main groups:

1. Directly related to cavitation
2. Unrelated or indirectly related to cavitation, namely:
   - Convection (the occurrence of acoustic flows resulting in the reduction of the boundary layer between the skin and the contact medium)
   - Thermal effects
   - Mechanical effects (radiation pressure effects)
   - Lipid extraction from the intercellular spaces of the *stratum corneum*

The key to understanding the mechanisms of sonophoresis was the discovery of the cavitation process — the formation of cavities (cavitation bubbles) in the liquid, filled with vapor of the liquid itself.

Although not all mechanisms contributing to the increase in skin permeability during sonophoresis are fully understood, it is generally accepted that acoustic cavitation (especially in the case of LFS) plays a major role. Acoustic cavitation is the process by which the following events occur:

1. Microscopic air bubbles present in the liquid increase in size or begin to pulsate (oscillate, i.e., expand/contract)
2. New gas bubbles are formed in the solution volume or around the crystallization centers
3. Any other type of enlargement, splitting, or interaction between gas bubbles resulting from acoustic oscillations in the solution is realized

In HFS with 1–3 MHz frequencies, cavitation is the primary mechanism for increasing skin permeability (Polat B.E. et al., 2011). The microscopic study conducted by Polat B.E. et al. (2011) revealed that cavitation occurs **inside the *stratum corneum*** in the spaces between the horny scales. This fact gives every reason to assume that oscillating bubbles directly affect the lipid barrier and change its structure, which leads to an increase in the *stratum corneum* permeability (**Fig. II-3-1**).

Under the LFS influence, much larger cavitation bubbles of 150 μm radius are formed. As this size prevents their formation in the *stratum corneum*, they instead form **in the contact medium**. Nonetheless, once these bubbles collapse, thin microjets appear (**Fig. II-3-2**) —

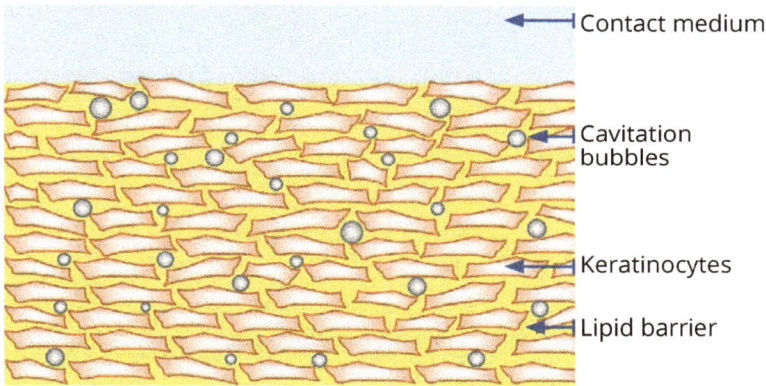

Figure II-3-1. Disturbance of the *stratum corneum* organization by the cavitation bubbles formed in the *stratum corneum* under the action of high-frequency ultrasound (adapted from Polat B.E. et al., 2011)

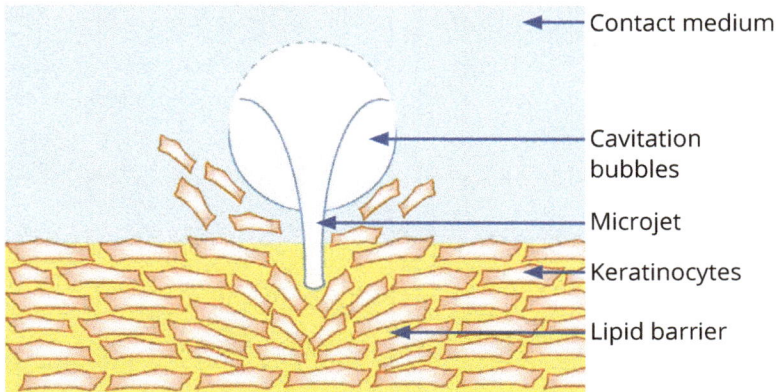

Figure II-3-2. Asymmetric collapse of a cavitation bubble with the formation of microjet near the *stratum corneum* under the action of low-frequency ultrasound (adapted from Polat B.E. et al., 2011)

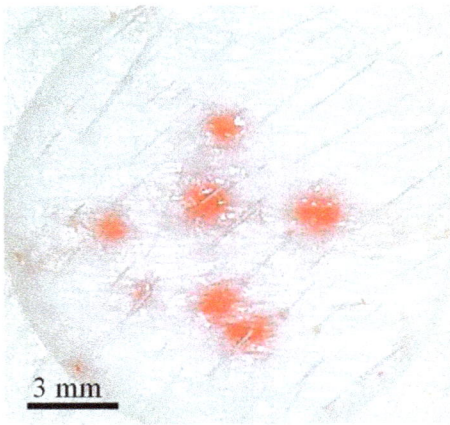

Figure II-3-3. Formation of localized transport sites (LTRs) on the surface of pig skin treated with low-frequency ultrasound (20 kHz) in the presence of surfactant. LTRs are stained with red dye (adapted from Polat B.E. et al., 2011)

they "hit" the *stratum corneum* with such force that lipids are literally "knocked out" from their intercellular spaces, leading to an increase in barrier permeability. Experimental evidence shows that during LFS (20 kHz, 15 W/cm^2), up to 30% of the *stratum corneum* lipids escape into the contact medium.

An important discovery in the field of LFS research was the detection of heterogeneous changes in skin tissue under the action of ultrasound. Namely, if the skin is treated with LFS (20 kHz, 15 W/cm^2), a single localized transport region (LTR) is formed directly under the ultrasound transmitter during exposure (**Fig. II-3-3**). In the LTR, the skin resistance declines by a factor of 5000 compared to intact skin. If a surfactant, such as 1% sodium lauryl sulfate, is added to the contact medium, multiple LTRs form on the skin surface during LFS exposure, and their total area can range from 5 to 25% of the treated skin surface. At higher ultrasound frequencies, transport through the skin occurs more uniformly over the entire surface without LTR formation. It is assumed that the collapse of cavitation bubbles with the formation of strong microjets "beating" on the *stratum corneum* is the most probable mechanism of LTR formation and skin permeability enhancement in LFS.

3.2. Peculiarities of the procedure

The ultrasonic hair removal procedure is carried out in two stages.

First, waxing is performed. Then, a special gel is applied to the skin before proceeding to the ultrasonic treatment. The gel is not only a sound-conducting medium, but also a carrier of active ingredients that inhibit the vital activity of HF cells. Proteolytic enzymes are used as active ingredients (see Part II, Ch. 4), along with other compounds that inhibit hair growth (e.g., *Narcissus tazetta* bulb extract, *Larrea tridentata* leaf extract, *Gymnema forestis* leaf extract, synthetic oligopeptides such as Oligopeptide-53 and CG-Nospotin).

The first qualitative changes are usually observed about 12 months after commencing the treatment.

Principle	The action of ultrasound increases the permeability of the *stratum corneum*, making it easier for active substances to pass through it and reach their target. The procedure should be repeated several times 3–5 weeks apart, as new hair grows back.
Advantages	• Relative painlessness (unless vaxing is poorly tolerated) • The ultrasonic technique of removing hair can be very effective when the particular hair unit is highly sensitive to the inhibitory effects of active ingredients
Disadvantages	The effect of reducing hair growth is achieved slowly
Complications	None noted
Results	The first qualitative changes are usually observed about 12 months after the first session

It is worth mentioning another technique once considered "true" ultrasonic hair removal. This technology was developed and patented by Applisonix (Israel) and implemented in the Selectif Pro device. The device is equipped with tweezers that capture the hair and transmit ultrasonic vibrations to it. In fact, the hair shaft serves as a conductor that transmits ultrasound energy directly to the hair follicle, causing heating and coagulation of the hair papilla. However, the selectivity of ultrasound conduction by the hair is questionable, as the ultrasound conductivity of skin and hair is about the same. This is confirmed by the relatively limited spread of the technology; despite being first discussed in the late 2000s, it was not widely distributed. Nevertheless, it has received considerable publicity, partly because of several lawsuits filed against the company. Nowadays, this technology has practically disappeared from the market.

The *Microcurrent, Ultrasound and LED Therapy in Cosmetic Dermatology & Skincare Practice* book provides more information about ultrasonic devices.

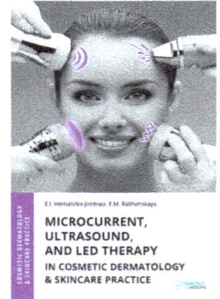

Chapter 4
Enzymatic hair removal

Proteolytic enzymes (papain, trypsin, chymotrypsin, elastase, etc.) that damage the hair follicle and cause its death can be used to remove hair.

Enzyme-based hair removal can be performed on hormone-independent areas, such as the lower legs, armpits, and bikini area. However, it is primarily used for removing hair in hormone-dependent areas, including the upper lip, cheeks, neck, chest, abdomen, buttocks, and arms. This technique can achieve up to 70% growth reduction for terminal hair and up to 90% for downy hair.

4.1. Mechanism of action

Proteolytic enzymes break down proteins, the basic building blocks of the hair shaft and the hair follicle (**Fig. II-4-1**). The difference between them lies in the mechanism and "potency" of action.

Papain is a hydrolytic enzyme found in all parts of the *Carica papaya* (except the roots), with the highest concentration found in the unripe fruit. Papain belongs to the class of cysteine proteases (which also includes well-known enzymes such as bromelain); however, it is the only one in this class that possesses exopeptidase activity, i.e., it "bites" the protein from the ends of the chain and can therefore degrade it to its original amino acids. The papain molecule has a mass of 20.7 kDa, making it a relatively small protein. However, even such a "modest" size significantly limits its penetration into the skin. Other enzymes have even larger sizes (trypsin — 24 kDa, chymotrypsin — 25 kDa). It should be noted that molecules with a mass of about 500 Da can penetrate through the *stratum corneum* without hindrance. Although

Peptide bond

R_1

O

H
N

Protein

N-terminus

N
H

C-terminus

O

R_2

H_2O | *Protease*

R_1

N-terminus

OH

Peptide 1

N
H

O

+

O

H_2N

C-terminus

Peptide 2

R_2

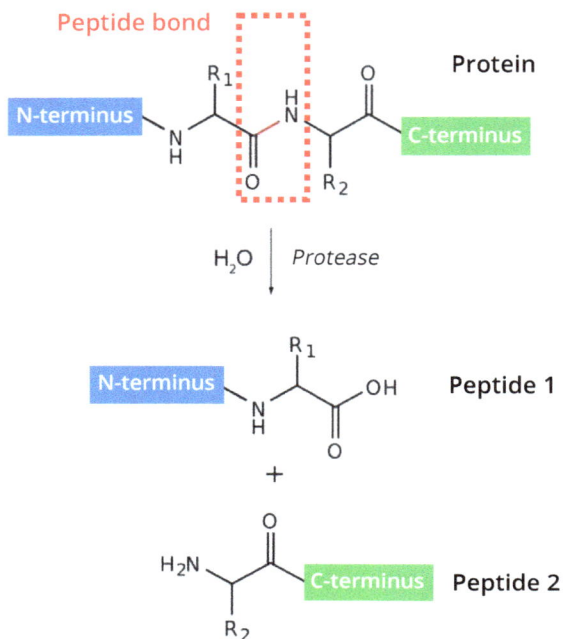

Figure II-4-1.
Hydrolysis of
a peptide bond
in a protein chain

the HF mouth acts as a kind of "elevator" through which larger molecules can penetrate and — which is essential in the case of epilation — reach hair follicles, the size remains too large. Thus, their "immersion" in the skin is achieved by destroying surface protein structures.

Studies in mice have demonstrated that enzymatic damage to the HF causes the detachment of its inner root sheath, cystic enlargement of the hair shaft, and a gradual decrease in the number of HF stem cells (Protopapa E.E. et al., 1999). Electrophoresis and liposome packaging were employed in this experiment to enhance the diffusion of the enzymes chymotrypsin and papain.

The type of enzyme preparation impacts efficacy. Traversa E. et al. (2007) evaluated histological changes in the skin and hair follicles of mice following the application of gel and cream containing papain (0.8%) using light microscopy. The tested preparations were applied daily to the backs of two groups of mice (10 individuals in each) for 31 days. Only 2 of the 10 mice treated with the gel exhibited a mild depilatory effect. In contrast, all 10 mice treated with the cream showed a pronounced depilatory impact. Notably, in both groups, the hair in the treatment area began to lose pigment and turned white. Histological analysis revealed no significant changes in the skin of mice treated with the gel. Meanwhile, thickening of the epidermis, a decrease in the number of follicles, and an expansion of hair bulb diameter by almost 55% were observed in the skin treated with the cream. The difference between the tested preparations was that the cream (emulsion) base contained an emulsifier — a substance that alters the structures of the lipid barrier of the *stratum corneum* and increases its permeability. This likely enabled papain from the cream to penetrate faster and in greater quantities through the *stratum corneum*, reaching its targets (stem cells, growth zone) in the hair follicle.

4.2. Peculiarities of the procedure

Human skin is thicker, and the HF depth is greater than that of mice. Therefore, the enzymatic hair removal procedure in humans is performed using methods that enhance skin permeability.

The treatment starts with cleansing and intensive moisturizing of the skin. If there is a lot of hair in the treatment area, it should be removed by waxing/sugaring or shaving. Next, the enzyme composition is applied, covered with a polyethylene film and heated with an IR lamp or a thermal bandage. In the heated area, microcirculation and metabolism are activated, and sweating is increased. As the occlusive polyethylene film prevents water evaporation, it accumulates in the *stratum corneum*. The bonds between corneocytes are weakened, the *stratum corneum* loosens, its permeability increases, and enzymes penetrate HFs more easily. The duration of the main stage depends on the treatment area, ranging from 10 to 60 minutes.

At the end of the procedure, a product with antiseptic, anti-inflammatory, and healing properties is applied.

Several treatments are required to achieve sustainable results, as it is usually not possible to destroy the HF in the first session. Procedures can be performed at any time of the year, every 30–40 days. There may be slight irritation during the first 2–3 sessions.

The enzymatic technique is primarily aimed at those who have a low pain tolerance and do not accept needle epilation. However, it is rarely used as a monotherapy and is usually combined with other hair removal techniques to prolong the effect.

Principle	Destructive effects of proteolytic enzymes on HF
Advantages	Relative painlessness (not considering the vaxing step)
	Ability to work in hormone-dependent areas
Disadvantages	Low speed of achieving an acceptable result
Complications	Individual reaction to specific ingredients
Results	Reduced hair growth

Chapter 5
Depilation techniques

5.1. Shaving

During shaving, hair is cut from the surface of the skin rather than removed, so the effect of clean skin does not last long, and in the case of thick, dark-colored hair, the skin does not appear clean because the remaining hair stumps are clearly visible. To facilitate the procedure and reduce skin irritation, it is recommended to use special shaving foams (**Fig. II-5-1**).

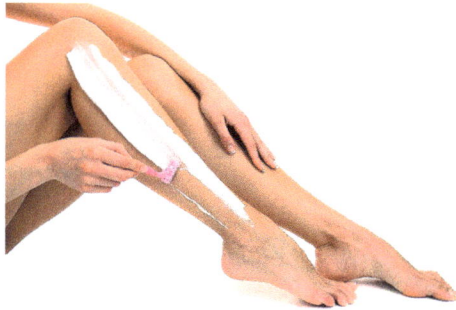

Figure II-5-1. Shaving hair with a simple razor

Constant shaving can make the hair darker, thicker, and coarser. Still, it is the most painless, quickest, and easiest way to do it, and no special skills are needed to perform the procedure.

5.2. Plucking or pulling (trimming)

Plucking hair with tweezers is a straightforward yet not very effective hair removal technique. Nevertheless, this technique is ideal for refining the shape of eyebrows or for removing individual hairs left after using other depilation techniques. There are various types of tweezers — with sharp, tapered, beveled edges, etc. (**Fig. II-5-2**). If the hair is pulled out quickly, it may break off; if pulled out slowly,

Principle	Cutting the hair that protrudes above the skin surface with a razor
Advantages	• Ease of implementation • Painlessness • Ability to eliminate hair in sensitive areas, including bikini and underarm areas • Expedience • Cheapness
Disadvantages	• Temporary effect • Hair ingrowth • Skin trauma • Irritation • Women should not shave facial skin due to possible stimulation of hair growth
Complications	Redness, sometimes irritation, ingrown hairs
Results	The effect lasts 1–2 days

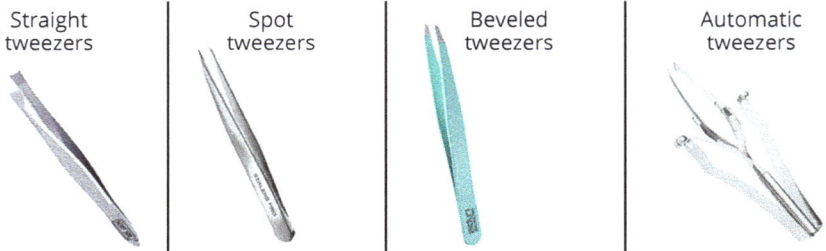

Straight tweezers   Spot tweezers   Beveled tweezers   Automatic tweezers

Figure II-5-2. Types of tweezers for hair plucking

the procedure can be painful. To minimize pain and trauma, the skin should be taut while plucking.

In addition to tweezers, a twisted coarse thread rolled over the skin is used for hair pulling — tall hair wound around the thread is pulled out. The advantage of this technique over tweezing is the ability to remove multiple hairs at once, as well as the convenience of working almost blindly by simply passing the thread over the skin. This technique is quite popular in Asian countries, but it has recently gained popularity in Europe as well — the thread allows for creating a clean line of hair removal, which is particularly sought after for eyebrow shaping (**Fig. II-5-3**).

The use of springs is a variation of the thread technique. When the spring is rolled across the skin, hairs are caught in the gaps between the metal spirals and pulled out (**Fig. II-5-4**). The springs also have the advantage of removing several hairs at the same time but can only be used for small hairs.

A more advanced variant of this approach is the use of depilatory devices that clamp and pull out several dozen hairs at once by rotating multiple pairs of plates or disks (**Fig. II-5-5**). As they rotate, they press tightly against each other, grabbing and pulling out hairs. Accordingly, all depilators are classified as either disk or tweezer (plate) type. To reduce pain, many manufacturers equip their devices with cooling, blowing, or vibration systems.

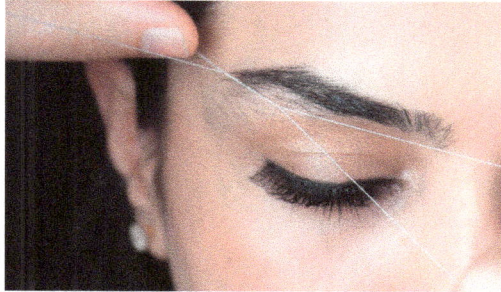

Figure II-5-3. Hair removal with thread

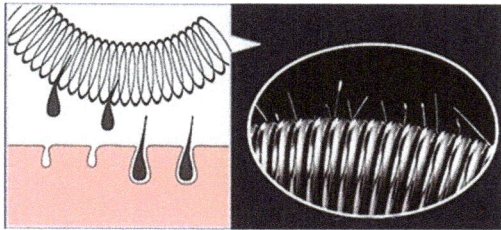

Figure II-5-4. Hair removal with a spring

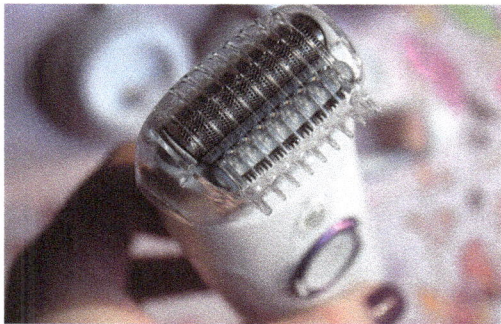

Figure II-5-5. Hair removal with a depilator

It should be noted that, in some cases, plucking hair (by various techniques) can lead to greater growth. Scientists have proposed that this paradoxical outcome results from HF traumatization during such mechanical action and the subsequent physiological healing response associated with the activation of blood flow and regenerative agents. However, it has long been unclear why this phenomenon occurs mainly after plucking but not waxing or sugaring. As part of their study, Chen C.C. et al. (2015) examined the molecular mechanisms behind this phenomenon in mice. It was found that HF injury causes the release of cytokines and an influx of macrophages, which, in turn, release tumor necrosis factor alpha (TNF-α) that stimulates HF activity, both in directly injured follicles and nearby ones. This phenomenon is called quorum sensing and serves as an example of intercellular communication, where some cells alert others to potential aggression and "ask" them to assist or replace them. Therefore, in the experiment, 200 plucked hairs were able to awaken about 1200 HFs both within and around the treatment area. However, the most interesting aspect of the study seems to be that the TNF-α "dosage" was critical for this effect to occur. Enhanced growth due to the activation of neighboring HFs occurred in response to plucking a sufficiently large number of hairs in a given area. This effect was not observed when only a few hairs or too many hairs were removed. Perhaps for sugaring or waxing, the stimuli are excessive or insufficient, thereby preventing the activation of hair growth.

Principle	Hair pulling with tweezers or a depilator device (clamping the hair in a spinning drum and pulling it out)
Advantages	• Ease of implementation • Expedience • Cheapness
Disadvantages	• Temporary effect • Painfulness, which limits the use of such techniques in sensitive areas
Complications	Redness, sometimes irritation, hair ingrowth, development of folliculitis
Results	The effect lasts for several days. Pulling a hair can damage the hair follicle, and constant traumatization of the follicle can eventually lead to its irreversible destruction. This explains the fact that, if hair is constantly pulled out, the amount of hair may gradually diminish.

However, it is much more common to observe a decrease in the number of hairs, along with their thinning and lightening, in areas where hair is frequently pulled. Histological examinations reveal changes in follicular morphology, including thickening of the basal membrane, a reduction in the amount of melanin, and an increase in the number of apoptotic cells of various types (keratinocytes, including in the bulge area, sebocytes). Microtrauma leads to transient changes in the expression of key components of neurogenic skin inflammation, thermoregulation, itching, and/or pain, which in turn inhibits regeneration (Bertolini M. et al., 2024).

5.3. Waxing and sugaring

Hair removal using wax and sugar molasses has been known since time immemorial and is widespread in Africa, Asia, and Europe. This technique remains very popular to this day, having gained significant traction after women's fashion became more revealing, especially with the advent of bikini swimsuits. In the 1980s, seven Brazilian sisters opened the first beauty salon where they began performing bikini waxing, which later became known as Brazilian waxing.

Nowadays, waxes for depilation contain liquid paraffin and natural resins (wood and synthetic). They are called warm waxes, as opposed to hard (hot) waxes based on pine resin or petroleum products that were used in the past. To make warm waxes easier to remove from the skin, a little sugar is added to their composition, increasing their solubility in water. Resin waxes are more challenging to wash off, and they must be removed with the help of oils. In fact, most wax formulations contain oils as they soften the skin and reduce irritation. When sugaring, thick sugar molasses combined with a small amount of lemon juice is applied to the skin.

The procedure steps are the same: the depilatory agent is applied, allowing time for it to bond with the hair shaft, and then the hair is pulled out with a sharp movement. However, wax is applied in the direction of hair growth and removed against it, while sugar paste is applied against the direction of hair growth and is removed with a reverse motion.

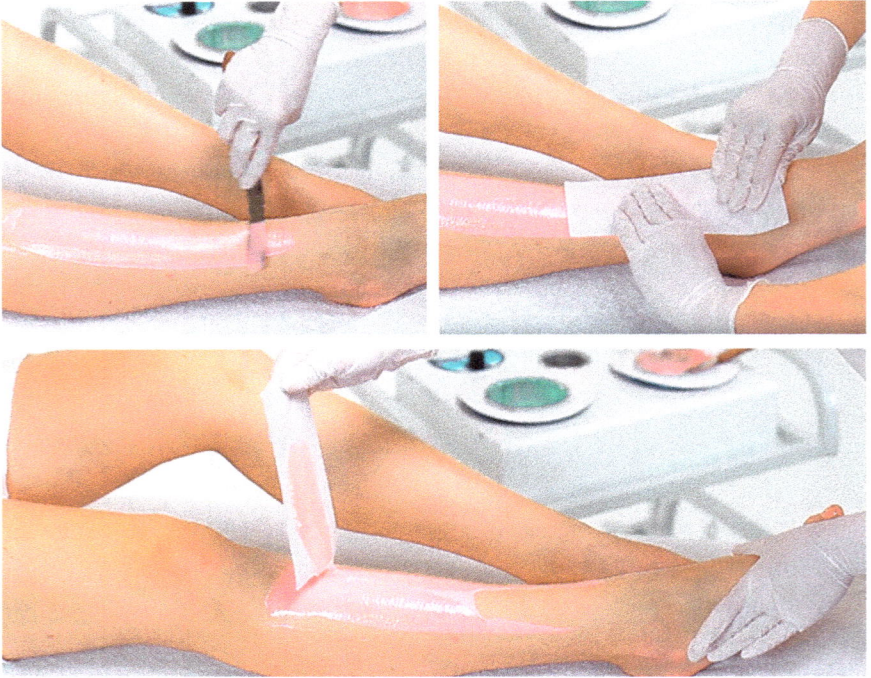

Figure II-5-6. Hair removal with wax

Wax and sugar pastes of different densities are used to treat various hair types. Thinner hair is usually treated with more liquid formulations, while thicker hair requires thicker formulations. Special cotton cloths are usually used to remove both waxes and sugar paste, but manual techniques can also be adopted (**Fig. II-5-6**).

Unfortunately, such procedures can lead to irritation, pain, skin swelling, and hair breakage (the latter is more typical for classic hot waxes heated to 42–60 °C). The modern generation of depilation waxes includes special polymer additives that lower the melting point and enhance wax distribution on the skin during application. Consequently, the wax no longer needs to be heated; it is sufficient to warm it under a stream of hot water or even in your hands. Cold waxes are heated to 35–40 °C and are commonly used to create coatings for special patches on cloth, paper, or polyethylene bases (**Fig. II-5-7**). Warm waxes are heated to 40–45 °C and are available in jars or special bottles with roller applicators (**Fig. II-5-8**).

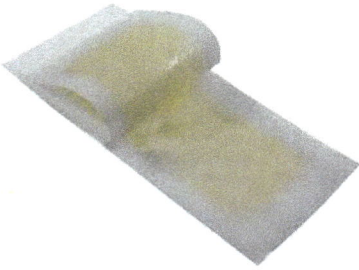

Figure II-5-7. Cold wax depilation strips

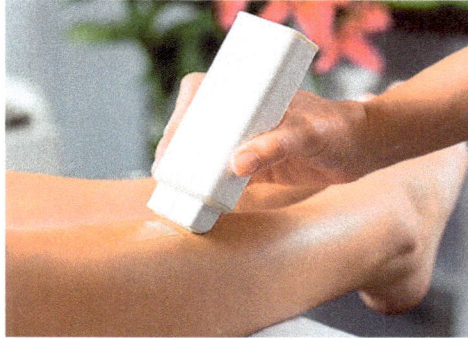

Figure II-5-8. Roller applicator for warm wax

The use of sugar is less painful because it captures the hair and the *stratum corneum* of the skin, while wax can also capture living epidermal cells, causing discomfort and irritation. Additionally, tearing off the depilatory agent in the direction of hair growth is less painful than against it. Modern ready-made sugar pastes are more malleable and safer than traditional ones, as they are made exclusively from sugars and do not contain citric acid, which may induce tanning. This technique effectively removes hair of all lengths and types, from fine to coarse, and even ingrown hairs (**Fig. II-5-9**).

Although both waxing and sugaring involve hair shaft pulling, the treatments can cause HF to break down, so the hair in the treatment area becomes thinner over time or becomes sparser.

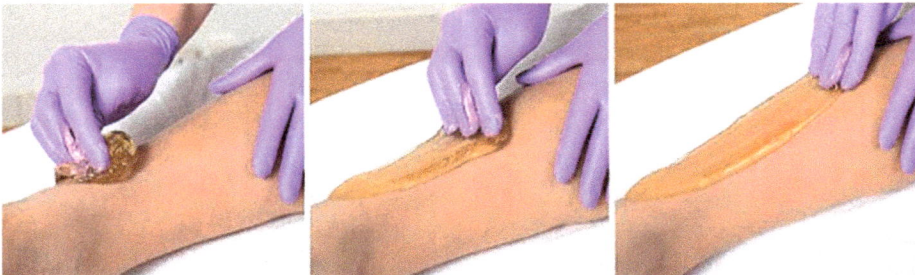

Figure II-5-9. Hair removal with sugar paste

Principle	Hair pulling with the help of a special adhesive composition: in waxing, heated wax is used, which hardens on the skin and is then removed together with the hair; in sugaring, a thick solution of sugar is used. Hair removal may be accompanied by HF destruction.
Advantages	• Relatively low cost compared to other hair removal techniques • Longer-lasting effect compared to shaving
Disadvantages	• Temporary effect • Pain (generally quite moderate), which limits the use of these techniques in sensitive areas • Burns may occur if hot wax is applied
Complications	Redness, sometimes irritation, hemorrhages, burns, hair ingrowth (more common with waxing than with sugaring)
Results	The effect lasts from a few days to a few weeks, then the hair starts to reappear. With prolonged and constant use of vaxing, the hair on the treated area becomes sparser, and its growth may slow down. It can be used in the intimate zone.

5.4. Chemical depilation and hair growth inhibition

Cosmetic depilation preparations can be divided into two groups:
1. Hair-dissolving (act on the hair shaft)
2. Hair growth-inhibiting (act on the hair follicle)

The first depilation formulations were invented in ancient India, where special creams were made from the juice of local plants. In Ancient Greece, women fought excess hair with bryonia root tincture. In the 15th century, the fashion for high foreheads and swan necks was widespread in Europe. To attain these beauty ideals, ladies shaved the hair above their foreheads and plucked their eyebrows, and to make their necks seem longer, they shaved the back of their heads. Then, to slow down hair growth, the shaved areas were covered with a mixture of vinegar and cat urine. Around the same time, even more toxic compositions based on arsenic and quicklime were sometimes used to remove hair from the body.

The prototypes of modern depilation compositions appeared in Europe in the late 1940s and quickly gained popularity. The main active components of these preparations were the same substances utilized for perming or straightening hair — thioglycolic acid, sodium thioglycolate, calcium hydroxide, sodium, or other salts of potassium, calcium, and lithium (which give a specific smell to the depilatory preparations, similar to the smell of perming agents). These compounds destroy disulfide bonds in the protein matrix of the hair, causing the hair to lose its structure due to which it "dissolves" and becomes soft, allowing it to be easily pulled out. The regrowing hair has a smoothed edge, which compares favorably with the sharp-edged spiky hair that remains after razor cutting.

The disadvantage of preparations that dissolve hair is an alkaline pH (11–12 on average), which is bad for the skin and often causes irritation. Therefore, when choosing a depilation product, preference should be given to preparations that have a lower pH value. It is also advisable not to leave the product on the skin for too long, as keratin is the foundation of the horny scales; when using the cream, the skin as well as the hair will be affected.

Various additives, such as anti-inflammatory extracts, vitamins, oils, etc., are added to depilation compositions to lessen their effect on the skin. In fact, it is these auxiliary ingredients that differentiate preparations of different brands, as the components that dissolve hair are mostly the same.

On average, the exposure time is 3–10 minutes, depending on the composition (for example, preparations with potassium thioglycolate act faster), and this is explicitly stated in the instructions for use. The cream is then removed either with a special spatula or rinsed off thoroughly (**Fig. II-5 10**). After depilation, hair begins to regrow after 4–5 days. The quality of depilation depends on the hair density and hardness — the thicker the hair,

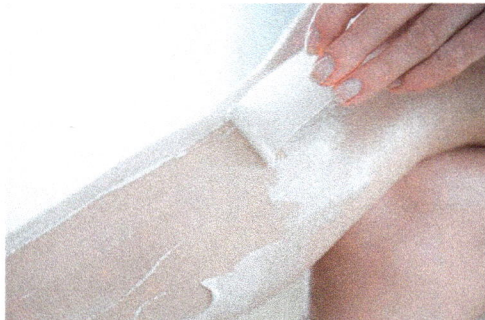

Figure II-5-10. Hair removal with a depilation cream

the longer the exposure time should be, increasing the risk of adverse skin reactions. It is therefore essential to carry out the procedures strictly according to the instructions.

Relatively recently, another category of depilators has emerged, focusing on the hair follicle. They contain substances that inhibit hair growth. Among natural ingredients, walnut shell extract possesses this property. There are also synthetic inhibitors of hair growth, such as eflornithine hydrochloride (included in the well-known Vaniqa and its analogue Eflora). This is the only drug confirmed by the FDA to be effective in stopping hair growth. Eflornithine hydrochloride blocks the enzyme ornithine decarboxylase, which is involved in cell migration, proliferation, and differentiation processes, leading to a significant slowdown, though not complete cessation, of hair growth. Its effectiveness can reach about 60%, which is not ideal but still relatively high.

Vaniqa is prescribed for women suffering from hirsutism and is recommended for use only on the face and chin. Since Vaniqa does not destroy the hair, but only slows down its growth, it does not substitute other removal techniques. Its effect becomes noticeable after 4–8 weeks of regular use and lasts for another 8 weeks after discontinuation. The most pronounced impact is noted with its continuous use for 6 months.

Principle	Use of special drugs that destroy hair shaft proteins (so-called hair dissolution) or inhibit hair growth
Advantages	• Painlessness • Can be used in sensitive areas • Longer-lasting effect compared to shaving
Disadvantages	• Temporary effect • Thick and dark hair is more difficult to remove • Possible adverse reactions to the product constituents
Complications	• Allergic reaction • Irritation (less common than after shaving or pulling)
Results	The duration of the effect and the time of onset depend on the product category

Chapter 6
Skincare after hair removal

General recommendations for skincare after hair removal:
- Only shower, no sponging, no rubbing
- Dry the skin with a soft, disposable towel
- Do not visit the swimming pool, bath, or sauna, avoid sports and fitness training during the day
- Apply antiseptics twice a day for 2–3 days
- Wear loose cotton underwear and blouses
- Do not use deodorants, antiperspirants, or alcohol-containing solutions for 2–3 days
- Do not expose the treated area to sun for 5–7 days, do not visit the solarium (after light-assisted hair removal for one month)

Hair removal using any of the techniques described here can traumatize the skin. To aid in its restoration, the cosmetic industry offers a variety of products — creams, sprays, lotions, gels, and wipes with special impregnation.

In general, skincare after waxing/depilation has several objectives:
- Restoration and strengthening of the *stratum corneum* barrier (vegetable oils, ceramides, silicone emollients)
- Deep moisturizing (amino acids, components of natural moisturizing factor) and surface moisturizing (hygroscopic polymers — polysaccharides, proteins)
- Skin cooling (menthol)
- Acceleration of healing (antioxidants, vitamins)

In addition, products that slow hair growth may be used (see Part II, section 5.4). If there is a risk of ingrowth, regular exfoliation of the epilation area is also recommended to help the hair to "break through" the *stratum corneum*.

It is also important to remember sun protection, as damaged skin becomes more sensitive to the sun's rays and can respond with hyper-pigmentation.

Part III

Common complications of hair removal

As with anything else, when removing unwanted hair by any means, it is better to take all necessary measures to prevent complications rather than to treat them. This is achieved through:

- Well-collected medical history
- Compliance with contraindications
- Taking into account the results of the previous procedure and skin phototype
- The right choice of hair removal technique
- Adherence to the technique and rules of the procedure
- Application of professional products before and after epilation
- Sun protection
- Personal hygiene
- Compliance with sanitary norms in the facility and the post-procedure skincare rules at home

However, complications after any type of hair removal can occur and can be categorized into several groups:

- Developing during or immediately after procedures
- Deferred
- Associated with existing diseases (both skin and systemic)

Foreseeable and unforeseeable complications can also be distinguished.

1.1. Complications that develop during or immediately after the session

1.1.1. Predictable complications

Predictable complications include the phenomena of **irritant contact dermatitis** — hyperemia, edema, and soreness (**Fig. III-1-1**). The common irritants in epilation are physical factors (exposure to high temperatures) and mechanical factors (removal of the hair shaft from the follicle).

Mild manifestations of irritant dermatitis almost always accompany salon procedures and are easy to predict. The intensity of these manifestations depends on individual skin sensitivity, hair thickness, the hair removal technique, session duration, and the technician's skills. Improper technique can lead to excessive pain, erythema, thermal burns, epidermal detachment, broken hairs, and hematomas. When performing hair removal independently, it is essential to follow the manufacturer's instructions carefully.

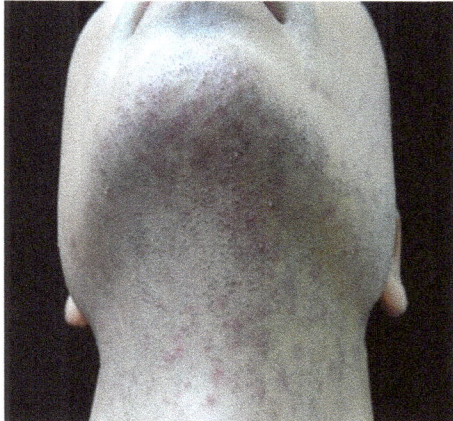

Figure III-1-1. Post-laser hair removal folliculitis (adapted from Juhong J., Tawanwongsri W., 2024)

Simple irritant dermatitis develops immediately and usually resolves within a few hours without affecting the person's general well-being.

1.1.2. Unforeseen complications

Unexpected complications may include **allergic contact dermatitis**, which develops due to sensitization to wax, chemical depilatories, and other substances used during the procedure. Skin damage occurs as a result of repeated exposure to irritants in individuals who are hypersensitive to these substances.

Allergic contact dermatitis does not develop in everyone, but only in sensitized individuals. Sensitization typically occurs after the first exposure, whereas during the second exposure, dermatitis appears immediately or within a few hours. Allergic contact dermatitis is more prevalent among individuals with a history of allergic skin reactions or those who suffered from atopic dermatitis in childhood, as well as among patients with eczema of any type, pollinosis, allergic rhinitis, conjunctivitis, or bronchial asthma. A well-collected history aids in preventing this condition.

The clinical picture of allergic dermatitis is characterized by erythema with indistinct boundaries, edema, and sometimes small vesicles, which, when opened, become wet and crusty (**Fig. III-1-2**). The rashes are accompanied by itching and burning. The main skin changes are concentrated in the axillae and in the areas closest to them, but due to the participation of the whole organism in the allergic reaction, they can also be observed at a considerable distance from the exposure site.

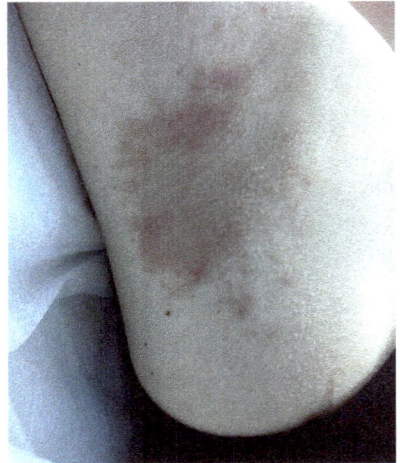

Figure III-1-2. Allergic contact dermatitis (photo by V.I. Albanova)

Allergic contact dermatitis differs from simple irritant dermatitis in that the severity of its manifestations does not depend on the strength of the irritant or the duration of exposure. Additionally, the area of inflammation is larger than the area of exposure, and the skin takes longer to return to its initial state after the irritant is withdrawn.

Complications such as **epidermal detachment** and **skin erosion** occur with waxing and sugaring if the procedure's instructions are not followed. A high level of expertise can therefore prevent both excessive pain and significant hyperemia.

If the skin is highly sensitive, the least traumatic hair removal technique must be chosen, including shaving. Chemical depilation is practically painless, but sensitive skin often reacts with dermatitis, so, as already mentioned, it is rarely used in the axillary area.

Folliculitis (**Fig. III-1-3**) is a purulent inflammation of the mouth of a sebaceous hair follicle and is the most common infectious complication of hair removal. Rashes in the form of single or multiple conical papules and pustules, infiltrated with or without hair, are located on a hyperemic base. These rashes are usually accompanied by pruritus and/or soreness.

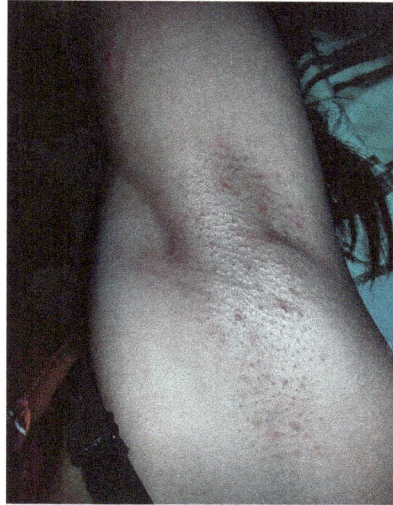

Figure III-1-3. Folliculitis (photo by V.I. Albanova)

1.2. Delayed complications

This group includes phenomena of microbial infection, such as folliculitis and furuncles, and subsequently emerging pathologies such as hair ingrowth and post-traumatic pigmentation.

Infectious complications such as folliculitis and furunculosis are more frequently observed after shaving at home or when skincare rules are not properly followed after salon procedures. Pustules, crusts, and skin damage prior to hair removal, sources of chronic infection like dental caries and chronic tonsillitis, diabetes mellitus, treatment with glucocorticosteroids, cytostatics, or antibiotics, as well as immunodeficiency, can serve as predisposing factors. The typical causative agent of these infectious complications is *Staphylococcus aureus*.

Furuncle (**Fig. III-1-4**) is a deeper lesion of the hair follicle area. Initially, it presents as a limited, large, painful, bright red infiltrate in the treatment area, but after 1–3 days, a pustule develops at the center of its surface. Once it opens, a considerable amount of white or yellowish pus is expelled from the resulting hole, and during healing, a scar surrounded by a zone of hyperpigmentation forms. These symptoms are accompanied by swelling of the axillary lymph nodes that lasts for approximately 2 weeks.

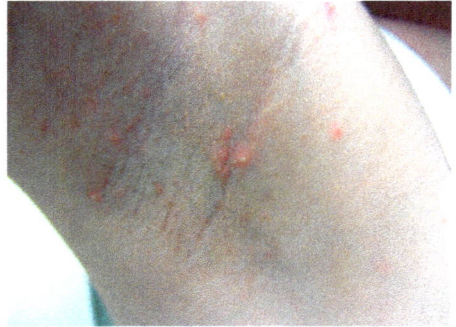

Figure III-1-4. Furuncle: bright red infiltrate with pustule formation in the axillary area after shaving at home (photo by V.I. Albanova)

Hair ingrowth can occur in individuals who frequently remove hair from areas covered by tight-fitting clothing. In this situation, the hair does not grow vertically or obliquely, but instead embeds into the *stratum corneum* of the epidermis. Perceived by the skin as a foreign body, the hair induces inflammation. A reddish-colored small nodule, where coiled hair can often be seen, frequently festers and develops into a pustule. These phenomena are typically accompanied by pain, moderate itching, discomfort, and a strong desire to pull out the ingrown hair.

Post-treatment pigmentation (**Fig. III-1-5**) typically occurs after light-assisted hair removal procedures and is often associated with frequent inflammation caused by hair removal. Post-session insolation and Fitzpatrick skin phototypes III–IV increase the risk of pigmentation. Axillary pigmentation is more likely to develop in obese women, individuals with diabetes mellitus, or those with

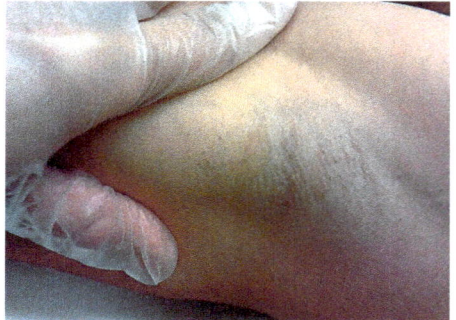

Figure III-1-5. Slightly expressed pigmentation of the axilla (photo by V.I. Albanova)

other hormonal disorders (**Fig. III-1-6**).

It is not uncommon for inexperienced practitioners to make mistakes such as incorrectly selecting application techniques, choosing excessive radiation density or wavelength, or failing to apply sufficient cooling to the skin. This usually results in inflammation with subsequent pigmentation or a direct stimulating effect on melanocytes.

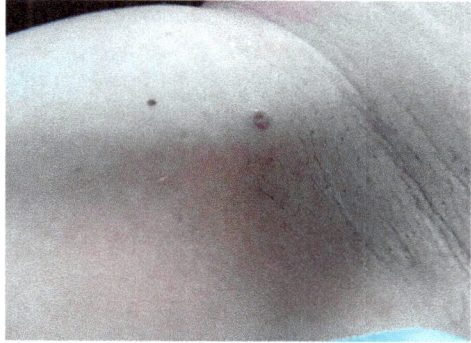

Figure III-1-6. Pigmentation in a woman with diabetes mellitus and obesity (photo by V.I. Albanova)

1.3. Complications related to existing diseases

This group includes exacerbations of chronic skin diseases (psoriasis, vitiligo, red squamous lichen planus), the spread of bacterial and viral infections already present before the procedure, increased clinical manifestations of dermatitis, diaper rash, and the growth of skin neoplasms. Even if there is no psoriasis, vitiligo, or red squamous lichen planus in the axillae, if it is present in other areas of the skin, there is a risk of new rashes in the areas of epilation — this is called Koebner's phenomenon.

In 1877, German dermatologist Heinrich Koebner first described a phenomenon in psoriasis known as the isomorphic reaction or **Koebner's phenomenon**: if a patient has active psoriasis, new rashes may appear on unaffected, traumatized skin.

Over time, it became clear that this phenomenon is also characteristic of certain other diseases and manifests not only due to mechanical skin trauma but also as a result of thermal or chemical exposure, shaving, vaccination, insect bites, surgical incisions, pruritic dermatoses, and other factors. The Koebner phenomenon can occur during hair removal (both mechanical and light-based), tattooing, microneedling, mesotherapy, and other invasive procedures.

There is a term "chronic koebnerization," meaning that rashes can also occur with chronic trauma. This is particularly relevant for delicate areas, as friction from the seams of tight clothing, which increases with sweating, is a common occurrence here. In connection with the above, it is essential not only to examine the site of future intervention but also to pay attention to the overall condition of the skin and collect a thorough anamnesis from the client. During periods of dermatosis exacerbation, salon cosmetic procedures should be postponed, and the client should be advised to neatly trim hair and wear loose clothing. The appearance of new rashes or an increase in the size of old ones is considered a sign of disease activity. At the same time, a stable course of chronic dermatoses allows for more active work in the axillary zone.

In viral infections, a reaction called pseudo-Koebner phenomenon is often observed, i.e., the appearance of new rashes around the traumatized skin of a patient with a viral infection. In this case, autoinoculation occurs, i.e., viruses are transferred by contact from one site to another. Viruses multiply well in the traumatized area because the skin barrier properties are compromised.

Mechanical damage to the skin during hair removal has been shown to cause sufficient trauma that can lead to the spread of rashes in diseases such as flat warts (papillomas), molluscum contagiosum, and herpes (**Fig. III-1-7**) (Sidharth S. et al., 2015).

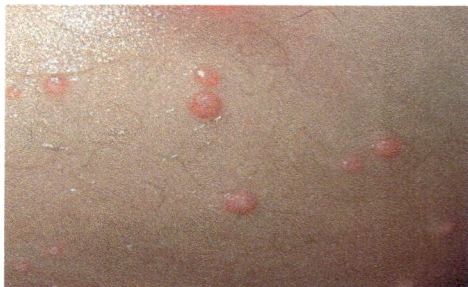

Figure III-1-7. Molluscum contagiosum in the axilla (photo by V.I. Albanova)

In addition to autoinoculation, infection from another patient is also possible, such as through the use of a shared towel, electric shaver, safety razor, or electric epilator. Attention should also be given to the treatment of instruments and materials (towels, sheets, tweezers, etc.) to avoid cross-contamination.

1.4. Treatment of complications

Skincare in case of complications includes daily warm showers with mild cleansers, drying with a disposable paper towel, and frequent underwear changes. To avoid transmission of infection, it is advisable to always have clean hands, short nails, clean and ironed bedding and underwear, etc.

Ingrown hairs with suppuration are treated as folliculitis. If there is no suppuration, exfoliation or scrubbing can help by removing the top layer of the *stratum corneum* and freeing the hair. Alternatively, the hair should be allowed to grow out, creating a loop that can be easily pried off with a needle to release the ingrown part. In cases of frequent hair ingrowth, using a scrub or hydroxy acid treatment before epilation is advised, and this treatment should be repeated several times with an interval of 2–3 days between sessions.

In dermatitis, cooling agents are used in the first hours, rest is recommended, and zinc suspension or baby powder can be applied 3–4 times daily. In erosions and blisters, cold lotions with manganese, lead water and furacilin, and diluted herbal tinctures (chamomile, calendula, etc.) should be used. In allergic dermatitis, external solutions of topical glucocorticosteroids (Elocom) are preferable; in case of severe itching, antihistamines of 2nd generation in tablet form (cetirizine, levocetirizine, loratadine, desloratadine, etc.) should be prescribed.

In cases of folliculitis and furuncles, it is essential to treat the entire area with antiseptics like chlorhexidine or 3% hydrogen peroxide. Then, solutions (e.g., Zerkalin), powders (e.g., Baneocin), antibiotic pastes (prescription medications such as erythromycin, levomycetin, lincomycin), or aerosols (e.g., Neomycin, Oxycort) should be applied directly to the lesions. For furuncles accompanied by a general feeling of illness and fever, as well as multiple bilateral pustular lesions, systemic antibiotics are prescribed: penicillinase-resistant penicillins (oxacillin, amoxicillin, flucloxacillin), cephalosporins (3rd and 4th generations), macrolides (josamycin, azithromycin), and fluoroquinolones (2nd generation).

In case of complications, trimming or using an electric trimmer is a preferred hair removal technique; however, it is better to postpone all treatments until recovery. If this is not possible, the affected area must be circumvented, and only disposable tools and materials should be used.

When treating the axillary area, the regional peculiarities of the skin — such as poor aeration, increased temperature, and humidity — should be considered. In local therapy, preference is given to solutions and powders, while creams are used less frequently, and ointments are never applied. Due to increased sweating in the axillary zone, occlusive substances are not advisable. Device-based physiotherapeutic treatment is also commonly used. Systemic therapy does not differ from the generally accepted modalities.

Afterword

Removal of unwanted hair is one of the most demanded tasks in modern aesthetic medicine. Nowadays, there are many tools available for this purpose, ranging from those that patients can use on their own, but with short-term effect, to high-tech modalities such as lasers and IPL devices that provide long-term hair removal but are only available in specialized salons. Their choice depends on the needs and capabilities of the patient, but also on the expertise and experience of the practitioner performing the procedure. Here, the higher the qualifications, the greater the chances of a truly long-lasting effect.

We hope that this book will help you appreciate all the intricacies of the task of removing unwanted hair, because only by understanding what exactly we are working with and what specific tools provide us, we can solve the problem in the best possible way.

References

Acle R., Zambrano-Mericq M.J., Navarrete-Dechent C. et al. Clinical and dermo-scopic evaluation of melanocytic nevi changes during diode laser hair removal: a prospective study. Lasers Surg Med 2022; 54: 970–977.

Adhikari M., Ali A., Kaushik N.K., Choi E.H. Perspective in Pigmentation Disorders. Comprehensive Clinical Plasma Medicine, 2018; 363–400.

Agrawal N.K. Management of hirsutism. Indian J Endocrinol Metab 2013; 17(Suppl 1): S77–S82.

Alajlan A., Shapiro J., Rivers J.K. et al. Paradoxical hypertrichosis after laser epila-tion. J Am Acad Dermatol 2005; 53(1): 85–88.

Altshuler G.B., Anderson R.R., Manstein D. et al. Extended theory of selective pho-tothermolysis. Lasers Surg Med 2001; 29(5): 416–432.

Andresen T., Lunden D., Drewes A.M., Arendt-Nielsen L. Pain sensitivity and ex-perimentally induced sensitisation in red haired females. Scandinavian J Pain 2011; 2(1): 3–6.

Ansari R.T., Syed U., Riaz M. et al. Unveiling the spectrum: a cross-sectional explo-ration of hirsutism causes in women. Pak J Med Sci 2024; 40(4): 736–740.

Arsiwala S.Z., Majid I.M. Methods to overcome poor responses and challenges of laser hair removal in dark skin. Indian J Dermatol Venereol Leprol 2019; 85(1): 3–9.

Aydin F., Pancar G.S., Senturk N., Bek Y. Axillary hair removal with 1064-nm Nd:YAG laser increases sweat production. Clin Exp Dermatol 2009; 35(6): 588–592.

Barbareschi M., Benetti F., Gaio E. et al. Capryloyl glycine and soy isoflavonoids in hypertrichosis: an experimental and placebo-controlled clinical study. J Cos-met Dermatol 2021; 20(Suppl 1): 18–22.

Bertolini M., Gherardini J., Chéret J. et al. Mechanical epilation exerts complex bio-logical effects on human hair follicles and perifollicular skin: an ex vivo study approach. Int J Cosmet Sci 2024; 46(2): 175–198.

Bhat Y.J., Bashir S., Nabi N., Hassan I. Laser treatment in hirsutism: an update. Dermatol Pract Concept 2020; 10(2): e2020048.

Bismuth K., Debbache J., Sommer L., Arnheiter H. Neural crest cell diversification and specification: melanocytes. In: Reference Module in Neuroscience and Biobehavioral Psychology. Stein J., Coen C., Rols E. et al. (eds.). Elsevier, 2017.

Bodendorf M.O., Wagner J.A., Grunewald S. et al. Efficacy and safety of laser shields to prevent radiant transmission onto pigmented nevi during laser epi-lation: an ex vivo histology study. Int J Hyperth 2013; 29(6): 539–543.

Boleira M., de Almeida Balassiano L.K., Jeunon T. Complete regression of a melanocytic nevus after epilation with diode laser therapy. Dermatol Pract Concept 2015; 5(2): 99–103.

Canat M.M., Erhan H., Turkkan C.Y. et al. Assessment of health-related quality of life in patients with idiopathic hirsutism compared to patients with polycystic ovary syndrome. Sisli Etfal Hastan Tip Bul 2023; 57(3): 332–338.

Chen C.C., Wang L., Plikus M.V. et al. Organ-level quorum sensing directs regeneration in hair stem cell populations. Cell 2015; 161(2): 277–290.

Coderch L., Alonso C., García M.T. et al. Hair lipid structure: effect of surfactants. Cosmetics 2023; 10(4): 107.

Cruz C.F., Costa C., Gomes A.C. et al. Human hair and the impact of cosmetic procedures: a review on cleansing and shape-modulating cosmetics. Cosmetics 2016; 3: 26.

Dessinioti C., Tsiakou A., Christodoulou A., Stratigos A.J. Clinical and dermoscopic findings of nevi after photoepilation: a review. Life (Basel) 2023; 13(9): 1832.

Drosner M., Adatto M. Photo-epilation: guidelines for care from the European Society for Laser Dermatology (ESLD). J Cosmet Laser Ther 2005; 7(1): 33–38.

Elosua-González M., Campos-Domínguez M., Bancalari D. et al. Omeprazole-induced hypertrichosis in two children. Pediatr Dermatol 2018; 35(4): e212–e214.

Elsaeed Eldeeb M., El Mulla K., Alshaer A. et al. The effect of long-pulsed 1064 nm Nd:YAG laser-assisted hair removal on some skin flora and pathogens: an in vivo study. Indian J Dermatol Venereol Leprol 2024; 90(5): 581–589.

Ezeh U., Huang A., Landay M., Azziz R. Long-term response of hirsutism and other hyperandrogenic symptoms to combination therapy in polycystic ovary syndrome. J Womens Health (Larchmt) 2018; 27(7): 892–902.

Fazel Z., Majidpour A., Behrangi E. et al. Using the hair removal laser in the axillary region and its effect on normal microbial flora. J Lasers Med Sci 2020; 11(3): 255–261.

Fernandes C., Medronho B., Alves L., Rasteiro M.G. On hair care physicochemistry: from structure and degradation to novel biobased conditioning agents. Polymers (Basel) 2023; 15(3): 608.

Fernandez-Flores A., Saeb-Lima M., Cassarino D.S. Histopathology of aging of the hair follicle. J Cutan Pathol 2019; 46(7): 508–519.

Finlay A.Y., Khan G.K. The Dermatology Life Quality Index: a simple practical measure for routine clinical use. Clin Exp Dermatol 1994; 19(3): 210–216.

Gacaferri Lumezi B., Goci A., Lokaj V. et al. Mixed form of hirsutism in an adolescent female and laser therapy. Iran Red Crescent Med J 2014; 16(6): e9410.

Garrido-Rios A.A., Munoz-Repeto I., Huerta-Brogeras M. et al. Dermoscopic changes in melanocytic nevi after depilation techniques. J Cosmet Laser Ther 2013; 15(2): 98–101.

Goel A., Rai K. Methods to overcome poor response and challenges of facial laser hair reduction. J Clin Aesthet Dermatol 2022; 15(6): 38–41.

Gold M.H., Weiss E., Biron J. Novel laser hair removal in all skin types. J Cosmet Dermatol 2023; 22(4): 1261–1265.

Guicciardi F., Ferreli C., Rongioletti F., Atzori L. Dermoscopic evaluation of melanocytic nevi changes after photo-epilation techniques: a prospective study. J Eur Acad Dermatol Venereol 2019; 33(5): 954–958.

Hinkel A.R., Lind R.W. Electrolysis, thermolysis and the blend: the principles and practice of permanent hair removal. Los Angeles, CA: Arroway, 1968.

Huang S., Kuri P., Aubert Y. et al. Lgr6 marks epidermal stem cells with a nerve-dependent role in wound re-epithelialization. Cell Stem Cell 2021; 28(9): 1582–1596.

Ibrahimi O.A., Avram M.M., Hanke C.W. et al. Laser hair removal. Dermatol Ther 2011; 24(1): 94–107.

Ibrahimi O.A., Kilmer S.L. Long-term clinical evaluation of a 800-nm long-pulsed diode laser with a large spot size and vacuum-assisted suction for hair removal. Dermatol Surg 2012; 38(6): 912–917.

James A.G., Austin C.J., Cox D.S. et al. Microbiological and biochemical origins of human axillary odour. FEMS Microbiol Ecol 2013; 83(3): 527–540.

Juhong J., Tawanwongsri W. Post-laser hair removal folliculitis: A case report. Electron J Gen Med 2024; 21(5): em606.

Kaliyadan F., AlTurki H.S., AlKhaldi R.D., Al-Dawsari N.A. Light-based home-use hair removal devices: a cross-sectional survey. Int J Trichology 2022; 14(1): 14–16.

Khurana K., Gaidhane S.A., Acharya S., Shetty N. Complex closed spinal dysraphism presenting as cauda equina syndrome with Faun tail nevus. Cureus 2023; 15(10): e47396.

Kim D.H., Lavoie A., Ratté G. et al. Effect of 27-MHz radiofrequency on hair follicles: histological evaluation of skin treated ex vivo. Dermatol Surg 2015; 41(4): 466–472.

Krasniqi A., McClurg D.P., Gillespie K.J., Rajpara S. Efficacy of lasers and light sources in long-term hair reduction: a systematic review. J Cosmet Laser Ther 2022; 24(1–5): 1–8.

Li K.N., Tumbar T. Hair follicle stem cells as a skin-organizing signaling center during adult homeostasis. EMBO J 2021; 40(11): e107135.

Lin X., Zhu L., He J. Morphogenesis, growth cycle and molecular regulation of hair follicles. Front Cell Dev Biol 2022; 10: 899095.

Mallat F., Chaaya C., Aoun M. et al. Adverse events of light-assisted hair removal: an updated review. J Cutan Med Surg 2023; 27(4): 375–387.

Marghoob A.A., Braun R. Proposal for a revised 2-step algorithm for the classification of lesions of the skin using dermoscopy. Arch Dermatol 2010; 146(4): 426–428.

Nabi N., Bhat Y.J., Dar U.K. et al. Comparative study of the clinico-trichoscopic response to treatment of hirsutism with long pulsed (1064 nm) Nd:YAG laser in idiopathic hirsutism and polycystic ovarian syndrome patients. Lasers Med Sci. 2022; 37(1): 545–553.

Nasimi M., Lajevardi V., Mahmoudi H. et al. Dermoscopic changes in melanocytic nevi following hair removal laser: a prospective study. J Cosmet Dermatol 2022; 21(2): 669–673.

Natarelli N., Gahoonia N., Sivamani R.K. Integrative and mechanistic approach to the hair growth cycle and hair loss. J Clin Med 2023; 12(3): 893.

Nishimura E.K., Granter S.R., Fisher D.E. Mechanisms of hair graying: incomplete melanocyte stem cell maintenance in the niche. Science 2005; 307(5710): 720–724.

Özyurt S., Çetinkaya G.S. Hypertrichosis of the malar areas and poliosis of the eyelashes caused by latanoprost. Actas Dermosifiliogr 2015; 106(1): 74–75.

Park S. Hair follicle morphogenesis during embryogenesis, neogenesis, and organogenesis. Front Cell Dev Biol 2022; 10: 933370.

Polat B.E., Hart D., Langer R., Blankschtein D. Ultrasound-mediated transdermal drug delivery: mechanisms, scope, and emerging trends. J Control Release. 2011; 152(3): 330–348.

Protopapa E.E., Gaissert H.., Xenakis A. et al. The effect of proteolytic enzymes on hair follicles of transgenic mice expressing the lac Z-protein in cells of the bulge region. J Eur Acad Dermatol Venereol 1999; 13(1): 28–35.

Puri N. Comparative study of diode laser versus neodymium-yttrium aluminum: garnet laser versus intense pulsed light for the treatment of hirsutism. J Cutan Aesthet Surg 2015; 8(2): 97–101.

Rafi S., Budania A., Bhardwaj A. et al. Efficacy and safety of diode laser for facial hair reduction in hirsutism — a clinico-trichoscopic evaluation. J Cutan Aesthet Surg. 2024;17(1): 19–24.

Raj Kirit E.P., Sivuni A., Ponugupati S., Gold M.H. Efficacy and safety of triple wavelength laser hair reduction in skin types IV to V. J Cosmet Dermatol 2021; 20(4): 1117–1123.

Rasheed A.I. Uncommonly reported side effects of hair removal by long-pulsed alexandrite laser. J Cosmet Dermatol 2009; 8(4): 267–274.

Robbins C.R. Chemical and physical behavior of human hair. 5th ed. New York, NY: Springer, 2012.

Sadick N.S. Combination radiofrequency and light energies: electro-optical synergy technology in esthetic medicine. Dermatol Surg 2005; 31(9 Pt 2): 1211–1217.

Sakina S., Behram F., Jadoon S.K. et al. Impact of laser therapy on the quality of life in women living with polycystic ovary syndrome-associated hirsutism: an observational study. Cureus 2024; 16(5): e61125.

Sari I.W., Kurniawati Y., Diba S. Comparison among intense pulsed light, alexandrite, and long-pulsed neodymium-doped yttrium aluminum garnet 1064 nm lasers for lower leg hair removal: case series. Int J Trichol 2023; 15(5): 197–203.

Sidharth S., Rahul A., Rashmi S. Cosmetic warts. Pseudo-koebnerization of warts after cosmetic procedures for hair removal. J Clin Aesthet Dermatol 2015; 8(7): 52–56.

Slee P.H., van der Waal R.I., Schagen van Leeuwen J.H. et al. Paraneoplastic hypertrichosis lanuginosa acquisita: uncommon or overlooked? Br J Dermatol 2007; 157(6): 1087–1092.

Soden C.E., Smith K., Skelton H. Histologic features seen in changing nevi after therapy with an 810 nm pulsed diode laser for hair removal in patients with dysplastic nevi. Int J Dermatol 2001; 40(8): 500–504.

Souza K.F., Andrade P.F.B.C., Cassia F.F. Castro M.C.R. Cyclosporine-induced childhood generalized hypertrichosis. An Bras Dermatol 2020; 95(3): 402–403.

Spritzer P.M., Marchesan L.B., Santos B.R., Fighera T.M. Hirsutism, normal androgens and diagnosis of PCOS. Diagnostics (Basel) 2022; 12(8): 1922.

Taylor D., Daulby A., Grimshaw S. et al. Characterization of the microflora of the human axilla. Int J Cosmet Sci 2003; 25(3): 137–145.

Thomas M.M., Houreld N.N. The "in's and outs" of laser hair removal: a mini review. J Cosmet Laser Ther 2019; 21(6): 316–322.

Torres F. Androgenetic, diffuse and senescent alopecia in men: practical evaluation and management. Curr Probl Dermatol 2015; 47: 33–44.

Town G., Bjerring P. Is paradoxical hair growth caused by low-level radiant exposure by home-use laser and intense pulsed light devices? J Cosmet Laser Ther 2016; 18(6): 355–362.

Town G., Botchkareva N.V., Uzunbajakava N.E. et al. Light-based home-use devices for hair removal: why do they work and how effective they are? Lasers Surg Med 2019; 51(6): 481–490.

Traversa E., Machado-Santelli G.M., Velasco, M.V.R. Histological evaluation of hair follicle due to papain's depilatory effect. Int J Pharmaceutics 2007; 335(1–2): 163–166.

Triana L., Palacios Huatuco R.M., Campilgio G., Liscano E. Trends in surgical and nonsurgical aesthetic procedures: a 14-year analysis of the International Society of Aesthetic Plastic Surgery — ISAPS. Aesthetic Plast Surg 2024; 48(20): 4217–4227.

Tsao H., Olazagasti J.M., Cordoro K.M. et al. Early detection of melanoma: reviewing the ABCDEs. J Am Acad Dermatol 2015; 72(4): 717–723.

Unluhizarci K., Hacioglu A., Taheri S. et al. Idiopathic hirsutism: is it really idiopathic or is it misnomer? World J Clin Cases 2023; 11(2): 292–298.

van Vlimmeren M.A.A., Raafs B., Westgate G. et al. Dose-response of human follicles during laser-based hair removal: ex vivo photoepilation model with classification system embracing morphological and histological features. Lasers Surg Med 2019; 51(8): 735–741.

Willey A., Torrontegui J., Azpiazu J., Landa N. Hair stimulation following laser and intense pulsed light photo-epilation: review of 543 cases and ways to manage it. Lasers Surg Med 2007; 39(4): 297–301.

Yamaguchi H., Funasaka Y., Saeki H. The effect of a frequency-doubled q-switched Nd:YAG laser on hairless mice harboring eumelanin and pheomelanin in the epidermis. J Nippon Med Sch 2019; 86(1): 27–31.

Yang F.C., Zhang Y., Rheinstädter M.C. The structure of people's hair. Peer J 2014; 2: e619.

Zonios G., Dimou A., Bassukas I. et al. Melanin absorption spectroscopy: new method for noninvasive skin investigation and melanoma detection. J Biomed Opt 2008; 13(1): 014017.

www.ingramcontent.com/pod-product-compliance
Lightning Source LLC
Chambersburg PA
CBHW052022030426
42335CB00026B/3248